2/83   1,950

D1127114

PRINCIPAL DRUGS

Principal Drugs

An Alphabetical Guide to Modern Therapeutic Agents

S. J. HOPKINS PhD, FPS

Consultant Pharmacist,
Addenbrooke's Hospital, Cambridge

FABER AND FABER
London · Boston

First published in 1958
by Faber and Faber Limited
3 Queen Square London WC1
Second edition 1964
Third edition 1969
Reprinted 1970
Fourth edition 1973
Reprinted 1975, 1976
Fifth edition 1977
Reprinted 1978
Sixth edition 1980 reprinted 1981
Seventh edition 1983
Printed in Great Britain
by Fletcher & Son Ltd, Norwich
All rights reserved

© *Sidney John Hopkins* 1983

British Library Cataloguing in Publication Data

Hopkins, S. J.
  Principal drugs.—7th ed.
  1. Drugs—Dictionaries   2. Drugs—
Nomenclature
  I. Title
  615'.10321   RS51

ISBN 0–571–18063–9

Contents

PREFACE TO SEVENTH EDITION   *page* 7

DRUG ADMINISTRATION AND
   RESPONSIBILITY   9

DRUG COMPLIANCE   11

WEIGHTS AND MEASURES   13

ABBREVIATIONS USED IN
   PRESCRIPTIONS   15

DICTIONARY OF DRUGS   19

APPROVED AND PROPRIETARY
   NAMES OF DRUGS   135

Preface to Seventh Edition

This edition follows the successful pattern followed in previous editions, and is designed to provide nurses and others interested in medicinal products and therapeutics with a concise guide to drugs in current use. A few old drugs have been retained where their use or interest warrants, but the emphasis is primarily on modern potent therapeutic agents. Most drugs are available under proprietary names, as well as under an 'approved' or non-proprietary name, and the latter is normally used in this book when a comment is made on the drug. Some prescribers prefer to use the 'approved' names in prescriptions, as recommended in the British National Formulary, but the practice is not followed exclusively. Accordingly, cross-references are provided from a proprietary name to the 'approved name', under which the drug is described, by the abbreviation *q.v.* (which see). To assist identification, reference can be made to the List of Approved and Proprietary Names on pages 135 to 186. In both parts of the List, a very brief indication of the nature or main use of the drug is given, and many drugs not referred to in the dictionary are included in the List. Some information on drugs merely listed in this way may often be found by reference in the dictionary to another drug of the same class.

An attempt has been made to indicate average adult doses, but this sometimes causes problems, as some drugs are used in different doses for different purposes. When a dose is expressed as a daily dose, that dose should normally be given as divided doses at intervals during the day. When a dose-range is indicated, a small initial dose should be increased slowly according to need and response. An indication is usually given when a drug is given as a single daily dose. For children and the elderly, lower doses are usually required. In the young, the ability to metabolise drugs may not be fully developed; in the elderly, impaired renal function may reduce elimination, and require a reduction in dose. For further information on these important aspects of drug use, standard books on drugs and pharmacology for nurses should be consulted.

My thanks are due to my former colleague, Mr D. B. McHutchison, BPharm, MPS, for valuable help and advice in the preparation of this seventh edition. Thanks are also due to those readers who have suggested improvements, and comments on any errors or omissions will be appreciated.

1982   S.J.H.

Drug Administration and Responsibility

Nurses should remember that the responsibility for drug administration is delegated to them by doctors, and that they act under medical direction. There is a trend to extend nurses' responsibilities to certain aspects of drug administration that are normally dealt with by medical staff, and nurses should be clearly aware for what they are accountable, and where their responsibility ends.

Before any drug is administered, the name of the drug and the dose should be checked with the prescription and the product. The golden rule is READ THE LABEL. If there is any doubt whatsoever, confirmation with a senior officer should be sought. **Belief** that the correct drug in the correct dose has been given is no substitute for certainty. Nurses are responsible for any errors that they may make, and must be prepared to accept the full consequences that may follow such errors.

Drug Compliance

An increasing problem of current therapy is patient compliance with prescribed treatment. It is easy for a doctor to prescribe, but to ensure that the patient takes the prescribed drugs in the right dose is a very different matter. The magnitude of the problem has increased with the rise in multiple therapy, and the reluctance on the part of some doctors to prescribe mixed products so that the number of different tablets or capsules to be taken daily can be reduced. It must be admitted that relatively few patients leave the consulting room with a clear idea of the nature and dose of the prescribed medication, partly as a result of fear of the doctor, and partly because of the difficulties of understanding complex therapy.

Here, nurses can play a valuable part in reducing difficulties and misunderstandings, particularly when dealing with the elderly and confused patient, and it is often helpful to ask a patient to repeat the directions that they believe that they have been given. Misunderstandings and errors can then be cleared up at an early stage. The containers of the dispensed medicines should not only bear the name of the drug, but also useful additional information such as 'The Heart Tablets' or 'The Water Tablets'. Vague directions should be avoided: whenever possible definite times for administration of drugs should be arranged. Such timing can be linked with some regular activity, such as a meal time, or a favourite TV programme may be used as a memory-aid for regular dosing. With multiple therapy, patients should be encouraged to set each day's dose aside, so that a double dose of a drug will not be taken by forgetfulness. Patients should be advised that the occasional missed dose is not always important, and a missed dose should never be made up by taking a double dose later on.

Although regular dosing is important in securing patient compliance, many modern drugs have relatively long half-lives so the regular administration of full doses for long periods may lead to overdose. The ideal dose depends on many factors, including absorption, metabolism, transport and excretion, but in many cases the margin of safety is fairly wide. In the elderly, however, reduced renal efficiency may lead to the gradual accumulation of a drug with insidious toxic effects. Many elderly patients, for example, on digoxin, may become over-digitalised because of poor metabolism and excretion of the drug. It is by no means unknown for elderly and confused patients, once admitted to hospital for observation, to make an apparently surprising recovery from an illness that was basically due to over-medication, often as a result of following blindly a misunderstood drug regimen. It is here that the community nurse has an exceptionally valuable part to play in ensuring regular and accurate medication, and reporting any incipient signs of overdose or side-effects.

Weights and Measures

Metric System

microgram (μg) or 0.001mg
milligram (mg) or 0.001g
centigram (cg) or 0.01g
decigram (dg) or 0.1g
gram (g). (In prescriptions the abbreviation
      'G' was formerly used, but is now
      obsolete.)
kilogram (kg) = 1000 grams

The metric measures of capacity which the nurse is likely to
meet are the
      millilitre (ml) which is approximately equal to the
      cubic centimetre (cc)
      litre (1) = 1000ml

Imperial System

(No longer used for prescriptions)

ounce (oz) = 437.5 grains
pound (lb) = 16 oz

ounce   = 480 minims
pint   = 20 fluid oz

Approximate Metric and Imperial equivalents

60mg	= 1 grain
1g	= 15 grains
28.4g	= 1oz
453g	= 1lb
1kg	= 2.2lb
63.5kg	= 10st
28.4ml	= 1fl.oz
100ml	= 3.5oz
500ml	= 17.5oz
568ml	= 1 pint
1000ml	= 35oz
(1 litre)	

Abbreviations Used in Prescriptions

The use of Latin abbreviations in prescription-writing is no longer recommended; the directions for use should be written in English, and in full. The use of some time-hallowed abbreviations still persists, and the following list is a selection of those terms that may be met with occasionally.

---

a.c.	ante cibum	before food
aq.	aqua	water
arg.	argentum	silver
b.d.	bis die	twice a day
c.	cum	with
collyr.	collyrium	eye lotion
crem.	cremor	cream
et	et	and
garg.	gargarisma	gargle
gtt.	guttae	drops
liq.	liquor	solution
lot.	lotio	lotion
mist.	mistura	mixture
mitt.	mitte	send
moll.	molle	soft
narist.	naristillae	nasal drops
neb.	nebula	spray
oculent.	oculentum	eye ointment
o.n.	omni nocte	every night
p.c.	post cibum	after food
p.r.n.	pro re nata	occasionally
pig.	pigmentum	paint
q.d.	quater die	four times a day
q.q.h.	quarta quaque hora	every four hours
q.s.	quantum sufficiat	sufficient

s.o.s.	*si opus sit*	when necessary
stat.	*statim*	at once
supp.	*suppositorium*	suppository
t.d.s.	*ter die sumendus*	to be taken three times a day
t.i.d.	*ter in die*	three times a day
ung.	*unguentum*	ointment

Note: The abbreviations s.c., i.m. and i.v. refer to subcutaneous, intramuscular and intravenous injections. It is usually made clear when a drug must be given by *slow* intravenous *infusion*.

DICTIONARY OF DRUGS

A

ACTH. Corticotrophin, *q.v.*

AT-10. An oily solution of dihydrotachysterol, *q.v.*

acebutolol. A beta-adrenoceptor blocking agent with a more cardio-selective action than propranolol and some associated drugs. It is therefore less likely to cause bronchospasm, and may be useful in asthmatic patients. Chiefly indicated in angina and cardiac arrhythmias. Dose 200mg twice daily, but larger doses may be required. Can be given intravenously in doses of 25mg in severe arrhythmias, repeated up to a total dose of 100mg.

acepifylline. A theophylline derivative resembling aminophylline, *q.v.*, but better tolerated both orally and by injection. Dose 0.5 to 1g three times a day orally, 500mg by injection, or 500mg as suppository.

acetarsol. An organic arsenic compound used in trichomonal vaginitis as pessaries of 250mg. Metronidazole, *q.v.*, is often preferred.

acetazolamide. A mild diuretic, but now used mainly in glaucoma. It decreases intra-ocular pressure by reducing the formation of aqueous humour. Dose, 250mg four times a day. Side-effects include drowsiness and tingling.

acetohexamide. An orally active hypoglycaemic drug similar in action to chlorpropamide, *q.v.* Mainly indicated in the middle-aged late-onset type of diabetes. Dose, 250mg increasing up to 1.5g daily as a single morning dose. Side-effects include gastro-intestinal disturbances, headache, skin rash and blood dyscrasias.

acetomenaphthone. An orally active synthetic vitamin K., *q.v.*, used in prothrombin deficiency. Dose 10 to 20mg daily. Menadiol, *q.v.*, or phytomenadione, *q.v.*, now preferred.

acetylcysteine. A mucolytic agent used to reduce the viscosity of pulmonary secretions in respiratory disorders. Used by direct instillation of a 20% solution in doses of 1 to 2ml hourly, or by nebulisation in doses of 2 to 5ml three or four times a day. Also of value in *early* paracetamol poisoning in an initial dose of 150mg/kg by slow i.v. injection, followed by smaller doses up to a total of 300mg/kg over 20 hours.

acetylsalicylic acid. Aspirin, *q.v.*

Achromycin. Tetracycline, *q.v.*

acriflavine. Orange-red dye with antiseptic properties.

Used as lotion 1:1000. Acriflavine emulsion is a bland application containing liquid paraffin.

acrosoxacin. A synthetic antibacterial agent highly active against gonorrhoea; often effective against penicillin-resistant strains. May cause drowsiness; care in poor renal or hepatic function. Dose 300mg as a single dose.

Actidil. Triprolidine, *q.v.*

actinomycin D. An antibiotic with cytostatic properties used in Wilms' tumour and tumours of the uterus and testes, and some bone tumours. Dose 0.5mg i.v. daily for five days. It also has immunosuppressive properties and has been used with azathioprine (*q.v.*) and other drugs in transplant surgery to reduce the risks of rejection. Great care is necessary in assessing dose and duration of treatment. Side-effects include bone marrow depression and alopecia.

Acupan. Nefopam *q.v.*

acyclovir. An antiviral agent with a highly selective action. It acts indirectly by inhibiting an enzyme essential for viral development and replication. At present it is used as a 3% ointment in herpes simplex keratitis, but may have wider applications. It is of low toxic-ity, and may prevent virus infections in patients receiving immunosuppressive drugs in transplant and cancer surgery.

Adalat. Nifedipine, *q.v.*

adrenaline. Known in the US as epinephrine, adrenaline is one of the principles of the medulla of the adrenal gland, but is now made synthetically. It acts on both the alpha and beta receptors of the sympathetic nervous system, and so simulates the stimulation of the sympathetic system generally. The effects on the alpha receptors result in vasoconstriction, with a rise in blood pressure, and stimulation of the beta receptors increases cardiac rate and output, and relaxes bronchial muscles. In acute asthma it is given as a 1:1000 solution in doses of 0.2 to 0.5ml by s.c. injection, repeated if necessary in 15 to 30 minutes. Doses of 0.25ml have been given by intra-cardiac injection in cardiac arrest and syncope. It is also used by s.c. and i.m. injection to relieve allergic conditions. It is added to local anaesthetic solutions (1:50 000–1:200 000) to prolong the anaesthetic effect by reducing diffusion of the anaesthetic solution. It may cause ventricular fibrillation if given during halothane, enflurane, methoxyflurane or trichloroethylene anaesthesia. In hypotensive crises, noradrenaline, *q.v.*, or metaraminol, *q.v.*, are preferred, as the intravenous use of adrenaline is potentially dangerous. Occasionally the solution is applied locally to stop capillary bleeding and epistaxis. Solutions of adrenaline may darken on storage and lose activity.

Adriamycin. Doxorubicin, *q.v.*

Aerosporin. Polymyxin, *q.v.*

Afrazine. Oxymetazoline, *q.v.*

Airbron. Acetylcysteine, *q.v.*

Akineton. Biperiden, *q.v.*

Albucid. Sulphacetamide, *q.v.*

alcohol (ethanol). Used occasionally by injection to destroy nerve tissue in the treatment of intractable trigeminal neuralgia. Industrial alcohol or methylated spirit contains 5% of wood naphtha; surgical spirit is industrial spirit with the addition of methyl salicylate and other substances and is used for skin preparation and the prevention of pressure sores. Coloured commercial methylated spirit contains pyridine, and is not suitable for medical purposes.

Alcopar. Bephenium, *q.v.*

alcuronium. A muscle relaxant similar to tubocurarine, *q.v.*, but more powerful. It causes less histamine release and consequent fall in blood pressure. Dose 10 to 15mg i.v., repeated as required with doses of 3 to 5mg. Reduced doses should be given during halothane, ether or cyclopropane anaesthesia.

Aldactone. Spironolactone, *q.v.*

Aldomet. Methyldopa, *q.v.*

aldosterone. The main mineralocorticoid hormone of the adrenal cortex. An excessive secretion of aldosterone may occur in some oedematous states and reduce the action of thiazide diuretics. See spironolactone.

Alevaire. A solution of tyloxapol, *q.v.*

alfacalcidol. A modified and very potent form of vitamin D, *q.v.*, but with a shorter duration of action. Valuable in vitamin D-resistant bone disorders. Dose 1 microgram daily.

Alkeran. Melphalan, *q.v.*

Allegron. Nortriptyline, *q.v.*

Alloferin. Alcuronium, *q.v.*

allopurinol. An enzyme inhibitor that blocks the formation of uric acid, and so is useful in the treatment of chronic gout. It also reduces the risk of uric acid calculi. Dose 200 to 400mg daily. Also useful in the hyperuricaemia of leukaemia. Side-effects include nausea, headache and pruritus.

Althesin. A steroid preparation of alphadolone and alphaxalone with anaesthetic properties when given by injection. Used for induction, or as the main anaesthetic for short operations. Dose 0.05 to 0.075ml per kg bodyweight by slow intravenous injection. The supplementary use of analgesics such as pethidine may be required. Bronchospasm and hypotension are occasional side-effects.

Aludrox. A gel preparation of aluminium hydroxide, *q.v.*

alum. Used for its astringent properties as a mouthwash and as a lotion, 1 to 2%.

aluminium. The powdered metal is used as a skin protective in ileostomy, as Baltimore paste, *q.v.*, also known as Compound Aluminium Paste.

aluminium hydroxide. An antacid with a prolonged action. Unlike the carbonates, it does not liberate carbon dioxide, is not absorbed and so does not cause alkalosis. Given in suspension as a gel (dose 7.5 to 15ml), or as tablets (500mg). Dose 1 to 2 tablets, chewed or crushed before swallowing.

Alupent. Orciprenaline, *q.v.*

amantadine. An antiviral drug, used in prophylaxis against some forms of influenza. It is also used in parkinsonism, and in association with other drugs such as levodopa, *q.v.*, may give valuable symptomatic relief. Dose 200mg daily.

Ambilhar. Niridazole, *q.v.*

amethocaine hydrochloride. Powerful local anaesthetic, used for anaesthesia of mucous membranes 1 to 2% solution; eye-drops 0.25 to 1%. As spray for throat before endoscopy etc., 0.5% solution may be used. Hypersensitivity and allergic reactions may occur as with other local anaesthetics.

amikacin. An antibiotic similar in actions and uses to kanamycin, *q.v.* Mainly used in the short-term treatment of serious infections due to Gram-negative organisms. Dose 15mg/kg daily (500mg twice daily in adults) up to a total treatment dose of 15g (adults). Side-effects include ototoxicity, drug fever, rash and nausea.

Amikin. Amikacin, *q.v.*

amiloride. A diuretic with an action on the distal tubule similar to that of spironolactone, *q.v.*, although it is not an inhibitor of aldosterone. It increases the excretion of sodium, but not potassium, and is used chiefly with a thiazide diuretic to obtain a more balanced response. Dose 5 to 20mg daily.

amino acids. Certain amino acids are essential for the formation of protein. When normal diets cannot be given, these amino acids can be given by intravenous infusion. Products in use may contain added glucose, alcohol and/or electrolytes. Representative products are Aminofusin, Perfusin, Synthamin and Vamin.

aminocaproic acid. An antifibrinolytic drug used to control haemorrhage due to excessive fibrinolysis. Used in major surgery and in the haematuria following prostatectomy and in menorrhagia. Dose 3g four to six times a day. Side-effects include nausea and dizziness.

aminophylline. Theophylline with ethylenediamine. It is more soluble than theophylline, but may cause gastric disturbance. It relaxes involuntary muscle, stimulates respiration and heart rate and increases diuresis. It is used mainly in congestive heart failure, asthma and cardiac and renal oedema. Useful by injection in Cheyne-Stokes breathing. Ampoules (intramuscular)

500mg in 2ml; ampoules (intravenous) 250mg in 10ml and suppositories of 360mg. Tablets (100mg) are available, but may be poorly tolerated. Some sustained-release products such as Phyllocontin are less irritant and better tolerated.

aminosalicylic acid. Sodium aminosalicylate, *q.v.*

amiodarone. An iodine-containing anti-arrhythmic agent of value in all types of paroxysmal tachycardia, especially when the condition is resistant to other drugs. Dose 200mg three times a day for a week or more for full response. Maintenance doses 200mg or less daily. Contra-indicated in bradycardia and thyroid disorders. May potentiate action of digoxin and anticoagulants.

amitriptyline. A tricyclic drug similar to imipramine, *q.v.*, but it has both antidepressant and mild tranquillising properties. Apart from causing some dryness of the mouth and drowsiness, it has few side-effects. Dose 30 to 150mg daily initially; maintenance doses 20 to 100mg daily. Lower doses often adequate in elderly patients. May be given by injection when necessary. Full benefit may not be obtained until after three to six weeks' treatment, and prolonged use may be necessary to prevent relapse. Contra-indicated in glaucoma, prostatic hypertrophy and pregnancy.

ammonium chloride. A mild expectorant and diuretic; has been given in association with mandelic acid, *q.v.*, in urinary infections. Dose 300mg to 2g.

Amoxil. Amoxycillin, *q.v.*

amoxycillin. A wide-range orally-active penicillin very similar to ampicillin, *q.v.*, but absorption is less influenced by food. Active against a wide range of organisms and is used in the treatment of respiratory, urinary and soft tissue infections. Dose 0.75 to 4.6g daily. Simple acute urinary infections sometimes treated with two doses of 3g, with a 12-hour interval between the doses.

amphetamine sulphate. A powerful central nervous system stimulant, but dependence may occur. It is now rarely prescribed except in long-acting products such as Durophet for obesity.

amphotericin. An antifungal antibiotic, effective in systemic as well as superficial infections. For systemic use it is given by intravenous infusion in a dose of 0.1 to 0.25mg per kg body-weight but reactions may be severe. It is used locally as lotion, cream or pessaries for candida infections.

ampicillin. An acid-stable and orally active penicillin with a range of activity similar to tetracycline, as it is effective against many Gram-negative as well as Gram-positive organisms (but it is inactivated by penicillinase-producing organisms). It is widely used in respiratory infections, chronic bronchitis and infections of the biliary and urinary tracts. Dose 250 to 500mg, six-hourly before meals. In gonorrhoea, a single dose of 2g with 1g of probenecid is given. Skin reactions are relatively common. The urticarial type is indicative of penicillin allergy, and requires a change of treatment; a macropapular rash is frequent with patients with infective mononucleosis and treatment with ampicillin should be discontinued.

amylobarbitone. A barbiturate of medium intensity. Dose 100 to 200mg. Sodium derivative is more rapid in action, but the effect less prolonged; it is occasionally given intravenously for the control of convulsions and in epilepsy.

Amytal. Amylobarbitone, *q.v.*

Anafranil. Clomipramine, *q.v.*

Anapolon. Oxymetholone, *q.v.*

ancrod. An anticoagulant obtained from the venom of a Malayan viper. It alters fibrinogen so that it does not react with thrombin to form fibrin, and any fibrin formed by other factors in the blood is rapidly removed by plasmin. The lower fibrinogen levels reduce blood viscosity, and the long action of ancrod is of value in deep vein thrombosis, retinal vein occlusion, embolism and vascular surgery. Dose 2 to 3 units/kg by intravenous infusion, repeated as needed.

Androcur. Cyproterone, *q.v.*

Anectine. Suxamethonium, *q.v.*

aneurine hydrochloride. Thiamine, *q.v.*

Anquil. Benperidol, *q.v.*

Antabuse. Disulfiram, *q.v.*

Antepar. Piperazine, *q.v.*

Anthisan. Mepyramine maleate, *q.v.*

antibiotics. Antibacterial substances which occur as by-products of the growth of certain moulds. The term now includes some synthetic derivatives of the natural products. The first to be discovered was penicillin, derived from *Penicillium notatum*. It remains the drug of choice in the treatment of many infections due to Gram-positive organisms, as it is highly effective against susceptible cocci, and is of low toxicity. Some penicillin derivatives (amoxycillin, *q.v.*, ampicillin, *q.v.*) have a wide range of activity; others (cloxacillin, *q.v.* and flucloxacillin, *q.v.*) are markedly effective against resistant staphylococci, and carbenicillin, *q.v.* is effective against *Pseudomonas aeruginosa*. Further research resulted in the discovery of antibiotics with a wider range of action, represented by aureomycin, chloramphenicol, the tetracyclines and the cephaloridine group of antibiotics. Gentamicin, kannamycin, amikacin and streptomycin, sometimes referred to as the aminoglycoside antibiotics, represent antibiotics used mainly in infections due to Gram-negative organisms, but are more toxic than the penicillins or related drugs. Streptomycin, *q.v.* and rifampicin, *q.v.*, represent antibiotics used mainly in tuberculosis. Wide range antibiotics should not be given for more than 5 to 10 days, as otherwise the normal bacterial flora of the intestines may be disturbed, leading to overgrowth of fungal organisms such as monilia.

Certain antibiotics

including neomycin and bacitracin, are too toxic for systemic use, but may be useful in the treatment of infected skin conditions.

A few antibiotics such as doxorubicin, *q.v.*, have cytostatic properties. Others, such as griseofulvin, *q.v.*, have only an antifungal action.

antihistamines. Drugs such as promethazine, *q.v.*, which antagonise the effects of released histamine. Of value in allergic states, hay fever, urticaria and other conditions where histamine-release is concerned.

antimony and potassium tartrate. Used in the tropical helminth diseases schistosomiasis and leishmaniasis. Dose 30mg by i.v. injection initially, increased slowly to 120mg, and to a total dose of 1.5g.

Antistine-Privine. A mixture of the anti-histamine antazoline and the long-acting vasoconstrictor naphazoline. Useful as a nasal spray to reduce congestion in rhinitis and sinusitis.

Antrypol. Suramin, *q.v.*

Anturan. Sulphinpyrazone, *q.v.*

apomorphine. A morphine derivative once used as a powerful emetic, but now considered too toxic.

Apresoline. Hydralazine, *q.v.*

Aprinox. Bendrofluazide, *q.v.*

aprotinin. An inactivator of pancreatic enzymes, used in pancreatitis and fibrinolytic haemorrhage. Dose 50 000 to 100 000 units intravenously.

Aquamox. Quinethazone, *q.v.*

arachis oil. Ground-nut or peanut oil. It has emollient properties, and is used in dermatology to soften the crusts of eczema and psoriasis, often in conjunction with calamine.

Aramine. Metaraminol, *q.v.*

Arfonad. Trimetaphan, *q.v.*

Artane. Benzhexol hydrochloride, *q.v.*

Arvin. Ancrod, *q.v.*

ascorbic acid (vitamin C). Present in many citrus fruits. Deficiency is unusual with normal diet, but a severe deficiency causes scurvy. Prophylactic dose 25 to 75mg daily; therapeutic dose 200 to 500mg daily.

aspirin. Acetylsalicylic acid. Widely used as a mild analgesic and anti-inflammatory agent, often in association with other drugs such as paracetamol and codeine. Dose 300mg to 1g, but in acute and chronic rheumatoid conditions doses of 4 to 8g daily have been given for long periods. Side-effects include gastric irritation with some blood loss, tinnitus and hyperventilation. The blood loss may cause anaemia if treatment is prolonged. Aspirin may also cause bronchospasm in asthmatic and other sensitive patients. Excessive and prolonged use may cause 'analgesic nephropathy'. Soluble aspirin tablets contain chalk to reduce the local irritant effects, and although a paediatric aspirin tablet is available, aspirin should not be given to children under one year of age. Aspirin may increase the effects of certain hypoglycaemic and anticoagulant drugs. The anti-inflammatory action has been ascribed to the inhibition of prostaglandin (q.v.) synthesis.

Atarax. Hydroxyzine, q.v.

atenolol. A beta-adrenoceptor blocking agent with the actions and uses of propranolol, q.v. Dose 100mg daily.

Atensine. Diazepam, q.v.

Ativan. Lorazepam, q.v.

Atromid-S. Clofibrate, q.v.

atropine. An alkaloid obtained from belladonna, hyoscyamus and other plants. Powerful antispasmodic, mydriatic, and central nervous system depressant. Often given by injection with morphine for pre-operative sedation and to reduce bronchial secretions. Useful in colic and peptic ulcer. Its use in ophthalmology to dilate the pupil requires care, as it may precipitate latent glaucoma. Contra-indicated in prostatic enlargement. The higher doses are given with neostigmine to reverse the muscle relaxant effects of tubocurarine, q.v., and related drugs. Dose 0.25 to 2mg.

atropine methonitrate. A less toxic derivative of atropine; used mainly in whooping cough and pylorospasm as Eumydrin. Also present as a bronchodilator in some inhalation products for asthma and hayfever.

Atrovent. Ipratropium, q.v.

Augmentin. A combined product containing clavulanic acid (q.v.) and amoxycillin (q.v.). Many penicillin-resistant organisms contain beta-lactamase in the cell wall, which inactivates penicillin before it can penetrate the bacterial cell and exert its toxic action. Clavulanic acid has no antibacterial properties but it can combine with the enzyme and inhibit its activity, and so allow the antibiotic to penetrate into the cell without loss of activity. This combined product has applications in the treatment of many hitherto penicillin-resistant infections, including some resistant to the action of beta-lactamase antibiotics. Dose 375mg three times a day, doubled in severe infections. Treatment should not be continued for more than 14 days. The preparation of an injectable form of the drug is under review.

Aureomycin. Chlortetracycline, *q.v.*

Aventyl. Nortriptyline, *q.v.*

Avloclor. Chloroquine, *q.v.*

Avomine. Derivative of promethazine, *q.v.*, used in travel sickness, nausea and vomiting. Dose 25 to 150mg daily.

azapropazone. A non-steroidal anti-inflammatory agent, with actions and uses similar to those of phenylbutazone, *q.v.* Dose 1 to 2g daily.

azatadine. An antihistamine with the actions and uses of promethazine, *q.v.* Dose 1mg twice daily.

azathioprine. A cytostatic agent that is slowly converted to mercaptopurine, *q.v.*, in the body. Of great value, in association with large doses of prednisone, as an immuno-suppressant in transplant surgery. Dose 2 to 5mg per kg daily. May depress bone marrow activity and care is necessary in hepatic dysfunction.

azlocillin. A broad-spectrum antibiotic with exceptional activity against *Pseudomonas*. Of value in respiratory and urinary infections, and in septicaemia. It is inactivated by penicillinase-producing organisms, but combined use with a penicillin of the cloxacillin type may increase the activity. Dose in life-threatening infections 5g by intravenous infusion eight-hourly. In less severe infections, 2g eight-hourly i.v. In patients with impaired renal function, doses should be given 12-hourly. Proportionate doses can be given to children. Duration of therapy 7 to 10 days. Allergy to penicillins or cephalosporins is a contra-indication.

B

BIPP. A mixture of bismuth subnitrate, iodoform, and liquid paraffin. Occasionally used as an antiseptic dressing, applied on gauze.

bacitracin. An antibiotic used by local application, often with neomycin, *q.v.*, in infected skin conditions. It is too toxic for systemic use.

baclofen. A muscle relaxant that acts on the spinal end of some motor neurones. Useful in multiple sclerosis and muscle spasms caused by spinal lesions. Dose 15mg daily initially, maintenance doses 40 to 60mg daily. Contra-indicated in epilepsy and psychiatric disorders.

Bactrim. Referred to under trimethoprim, q.v.

Baltimore paste. Compound Aluminium Paste B.P.C. Contains aluminium powder, zinc oxide and liquid paraffin. It is used as a skin protective in ileostomy and similar conditions.

bamethan. A peripheral vasodilator used in circulatory disorders such as Raynaud's disease, and leg ulcers. Dose 100mg daily.

Banistyl. Dimethothiazine, q.v.

Banocide. Diethylcarbamazine, q.v.

Baratol. Indoramin, q.v.

barbiturates. A group of hypnotic drugs exemplified by butobarbitone, q.v. Once widely used, but their value has declined sharply as safer drugs such as nitrazepam, q.v. have been introduced.

barium sulphate. A very insoluble powder, given orally or rectally as an aqueous suspension as contrast agent for x-ray examination of the alimentary system. *Note: Soluble* salts of barium are very poisonous.

Baycaron. Mefruside, q.v.

Baypen. Mezlocillin, q.v.

beclamide. An anticonvulsant used in grand mal and psychomotor epilepsy. May be given in association with phenobarbitone. Dose 0.5 to 1g, three to four times a day.

beclomethasone. A potent corticosteroid for local application. Used as ointment or cream (0.025%), often with neomycin; by oral inhalation in asthma, and as nasal aerosol for hayfever.

Beconase. A preparation of beclomethasone for use in hayfever.

Becotide. A preparation of beclomethasone, q.v., for oral inhalation in the treatment of asthma. May permit the reduction in dose of systemic steroids.

belladonna. The deadly nightshade (*Atropa belladonna*). The principal constituent is atropine, q.v.

bemegride. A respiratory stimulant used occasionally in barbiturate intoxication. Dose 50mg i.v. repeated at intervals of three to five minutes according to response.

Benadon. Pyridoxine, q.v.

Benadryl. Diphenhydramine, q.v.

bendrofluazide. A diuretic of the chlorothiazide type, but with a more powerful and prolonged action. Used in congestive heart failure, oedema, and in hypertension to potentiate the action of antihypertensive drugs. Potassium supplements are necessary with prolonged treatment. Dose 2.5 to 10mg daily.

Benemid. Probenecid, *q.v.*

Benerva. Thiamine hydrochloride, *q.v.*

Benoral. Benorylate, *q.v.*

benorylate. A derivative of aspirin and paracetamol, with the general properties of both drugs. Used in arthritic conditions and for the relief of painful musculoskeletal disorders. Like aspirin, it may cause gastro-intestinal disturbances and increase the action of oral anticoagulants. Dose 1 to 2g four times a day.

benoxaprofen. A non-steroidal anti-inflammatory agent for the relief of rheumatoid and osteoarthritis. Causes less gastric disturbance than related drugs. Effective in a single dose of 600mg daily at night, or as 300mg twice daily. Care advised in hepatic dysfunction; photosensitive skin reactions have occurred.

benperidol. A tranquilliser for use in controlling antisocial sexual behaviour. Dose 0.25 to 1.5mg daily.

benserazide. An enzyme inhibitor used with levodopa, *q.v.*, in parkinsonism. It prevents the breakdown of levodopa, thus permitting a larger amount to reach the brain.

benzalkonium chloride. A detergent with antiseptic properties present in various skin preparations.

benzathine penicillin. A long-acting penicillin compound; present in Penidural.

benzhexol hydrochloride. A spasmolytic drug with atropine-like properties used mainly to relieve the tremor and rigidity of parkinsonism. Initial doses should be small, increased gradually until the optimum effect is obtained. Side-effects include dry mouth, and psychiatric disturbances may require cessation of use. Dose 2 to 20mg daily.

benzocaine. A local anaesthetic for topical application. Used as lozenges (100mg) for painful oral conditions; ointment (5 to 10%); suppositories 200mg.

benzoctamine. A minor tranquilliser used in anxiety and tension states. Dose 10 to 20mg three times a day.

benzoic acid. It has fungistatic properties similar to salicylic acid, and is used as Whitfield's ointment (Compound Benzoic Acid Ointment) for the treatment of ringworm.

benzoin. A balsamic resin used in the treatment of bronchitis, pharyngitis and catarrh by steam inhalation of friar's balsam (Compound Tincture of Benzoin).

benzoyl peroxide. A locally acting agent, often used in association with sulphur, as a cream or gel in acne.

benzthiazide. A diuretic present with triamterene, *q.v*, in Dytide.

benztropine. A spasmolytic drug used to relieve the rigidity, muscle spasm, tremor and salivation of Parkinson's disease. It has some sedative action, and may be preferred to benzhexol, *q.v.* Dose 0.5 to 6mg daily.

benzyl benzoate. A clear liquid with an aromatic odour. It is used as an emulsion in the treatment of scabies by two applications to the whole of the body except the head.

benzyl penicillin. Penicillin, *q.v.*

bephenium. An anthelmintic effective against hookworm and roundworm. Given as a single dose of 5g on an empty stomach. A second dose may be given later if necessary.

Berotec. Fenoterol, *q.v.*

beta-adrenergic blocking agents. Adrenaline and related catecholamines are released into the circulation during exercise and stress, and stimulate cardiac output by acting on the beta-adrenoreceptor sites in the heart. When such stimulation is excessive the increased oxygen demand of the heart may cause myocardial insufficiency and angina. Drugs such as propranolol, *q.v*, block these receptor sites and so indirectly reduce cardiac stimulation, and are of value in the control of angina. Some blocking agents also act on other receptor sites and may cause bronchospasm by releasing histamine. Newer drugs, represented by acebutolol, *q.v.*, and metoprolol, are more cardioselective, and others such as sotalol, *q.v.*, are of more value in hypertension. By the nature of these drugs, care is necessary in heart block and cardiogenic shock.

Beta-Cardone. Sotalol, *q.v.*

Betadine. Povidone-iodine, *q.v.*

betahistine. A vasodilator with some of the properties of histamine. Used to reduce the vertigo of Ménière's disease. Should be used with care in asthmatics. Dose 8 to 48mg daily.

Betaloc. Metoprolol, *q.v.*

betamethasone. A synthetic corticosteroid characterised by the low dose, increased anti-inflammatory action, and reduced side-effects. It has virtually no salt-retaining properties, and causes little increase in the urinary excretion of potassium. Indicated in all conditions requiring corticosteroid therapy, with the exception of Addison's disease and after adrenalectomy when a salt-retaining steroid is required. Dose 0.5 to 5mg daily in divided doses. Preparations for topical use are also available.

bethanechol. A parasympathomimetic agent used in gastric and intestinal retention, and postoperative urinary retention. Dose 5 to 30mg three or four times a day before food.

bethanidine. An antihypertensive agent that functions by a selective action on postganglionic adrenergic nerves, inhibiting the release of noradrenaline. Useful in severe hypertension, or when guanethidine or related drugs are not well tolerated. Dose 20 to 200mg daily.

Betnelan. Betamethasone, *q.v.*

Betnovate. Skin preparations of betamethasone, *q.v.*

BICNU. Carmustine, *q.v.*

Biligrafin. A radio-opaque diagnostic agent. Given by intravenous injection for x-ray visualisation of the biliary tract.

Biogastrone. Carbenoxolone, *q.v.*

Bioral. Carbenoxolone, *q.v.*

biperiden. An antispasmodic and parasympatholytic drug, used chiefly to control the rigidity and excessive salivation of parkinsonism. It has less effect on tremor. Dose 1 to 2mg, increased as required up to 12mg daily.

bisacodyl. A synthetic laxative that exerts its action by a direct stimulating effect on the nerve endings of the colon. Dose 10mg orally, or as a suppository.

bismuth subgallate. A yellow insoluble powder with astringent properties. Used as dusting powder, and as suppositories for rectal conditions.

bismuth subnitrate. A constituent of BIPP, *q.v.*

Bisolvon. Bromhexine, *q.v.*

bleomycin. An antibiotic with cytotoxic properties. Exceptional in causing little if any disturbance of bone marrow activity. Used mainly in skin tumours, lymphomas, and mycosis fungoides. Dose 15 to 30mg twice-weekly by i.m. or i.v. injection up to a total dose of 300mg.

Blocadren. Timolol, *q.v.*

Bolvidon. Mianserin, *q.v.*

boric acid, boracic acid. Mild antiseptic. Should not be applied to large, raw areas owing to risk of absorption in toxic amounts.

Bradilan. Nicofuranose, *q.v.*

Bradosol. Domiphen, *q.v.*

Breoprin. Aspirin, q.v.

Bretylate. Bretylium, q.v.

bretylium. An antihypertensive agent, but less reliable than guanethidine, q.v. Used mainly in the control of resistant ventricular arrhythmias. Dose 5mg/kg, i.m., 6- to 8-hourly.

Brevidil. Suxamethonium, q.v.

Bricanyl. Terbutaline, q.v.

Brietal. Methohexitone, q.v.

brilliant green. An antiseptic dye occasionally used as a lotion, 1 in 1000; also as an ointment (2%).

Brinaldix. Clopamide, q.v.

Brocadopa. Levodopa, q.v.

bromhexine. An expectorant with mucolytic properties. It stimulates the production of thin, easily expectorated sputum. Useful in acute and chronic bronchitis when tenacious sputum complicates treatment. Dose 24 to 64mg daily.

bromocriptine. A therapeutic agent with a selective action on the pituitary gland. It is used for the inhibition of lactation, but may have wider applications in other conditions associated with pituitary dysfunction such as acromegaly, parkinsonism and mastalgia. Treatment is gradual, beginning with 1.25 to 2.5mg daily, increasing according to need and response, which in acromeg-

aly may be as high as 60mg daily.

brompheniramine. An antihistamine similar to promethazine, q.v., but with a shorter action and less side-effects. It also has some antitussive properties. Dose 12 to 32mg daily.

Broxil. Phenethicillin, q.v.

Brufen. Ibuprofen, q.v.

bumetanide. A diuretic similar to frusemide, q.v. Dose 1 to 5mg daily. In acute pulmonary and cardiac oedema, doses of 1 to 2mg may be given intravenously.

bupivacaine. A local anaesthetic related to lignocaine, but characterised by its increased potency and long duration of action. Used as a 0.25 to 0.5% solution, with or without adrenaline.

buprenorphine. A powerful analgesic, related to morphine, but less likely to cause dependence. Valuable in pain of terminal cancer, after operation or myocardial infarction. Care necessary in respiratory depression or hepatic disease. Dose 0.3 to 0.6mg by i.m. or slow intravenous infusion at intervals of six to eight hours.

Burinex. Bumetanide, q.v.

Buscopan. Hyoscine butylbromide, q.v.

busulphan. A cytostatic compound used in the palliative

treatment of chronic myeloid leukaemia. Close haematological control is essential during treatment as remission of symptoms may not be complete for some weeks. Dose 0.5 to 4mg daily.

Butacote. Phenylbutazone, *q.v.*

Butazolidin. Phenylbutazone, *q.v.*

butobarbitone. A barbiturate of medium intensity and rapidity of onset. Dose 60 to 200mg.

butorphanol. An analgesic similar to buprenorphine, *q.v.* Dose 1mg i.v. or 2mg i.m. three- to four-hourly.

C

CCNU. Lomustine, *q.v.*

cade oil. An old treatment for psoriasis and some forms of eczema. Used as ointment and shampoo, and as medicated soap for seborrhoea.

caffeine. The central nervous system stimulant present in tea and coffee. It is used with paracetamol and other mild analgesics. Dose 100 to 300mg. Caffeine sodium benzoate is a soluble compound used by injection as a cardiac and respiratory stimulant. Dose 0.3 to 1g.

calamine. Zinc carbonate. It has a mild astringent and soothing action when applied to the skin, and is widely used as Calamine Lotion for skin

irritation and as Oily Calamine Lotion in eczema.

calciferol (vitamin D_2). The form of vitamin D, *q.v.*, used in the prophylaxis and treatment of deficiency states such as rickets in children and osteomalacia in adults, and in other bone disorders. Prophylactic dose 800 units daily, therapeutic dose 5000 to 50 000 units daily. In resistant rickets and parathyroid deficiency, higher doses may be required, but such therapy requires care, as hypercalcaemia and irreversible renal damage may occur.

Calcitare. Calcitonin, *q.v.*

calcitonin. A hormone of the thyroid gland, which has an action similar to that of the parathyroid gland in regulating blood calcium levels. Given in the hypercalcaemia due to tumours, in osteoporosis, and in Paget's disease. Dose may vary from 10 to 160 units daily by injection.

Calciparine. The calcium salt of heparin, *q.v.*

calcitriol. One of the most powerful metabolites of vitamin D, *q.v.* Used in renal osteodystrophy. Dose 1 to 3 micrograms daily.

calcium carbonate. Chalk, *q.v.*

calcium chloride. Has the general action of calcium salts but because of its irritant side-effects, calcium gluconate, *q.v.*, is usually preferred.

calcium gluconate. A soluble and well-tolerated calcium salt used in many conditions associated with calcium deficiency such as tetany, rickets, coeliac disease, parathyroid deficiency; also during pregnancy and lactation often in association with vitamin D. Calcium gluconate is also given in chilblains, urticaria and allergic reactions. The drug may be given orally, intramuscularly as a 10% solution, or in emergency by slow intravenous injection. Dose 1 to 5g.

calcium lactate. Given in calcium-deficiency states, but calcium gluconate is usually preferred. Dose 1 to 5g.

Calcium Resonium. An ion-exchange resin that takes up potassium in exchange for calcium. Used in hyperkalaemia associated with anuria and haemodialysis. Should be used only when potassium and calcium serum levels are under biochemical control. Dose 15 to 30g three or four times a day. For children, 0.5 to 1g/kg daily.

Calpol. Paracetamol, *q.v.*

Calsynar. Salcatonin, *q.v.*

Calthor. Ciclacillin, *q.v.*

Camcolit. Lithium carbonate, *q.v.*

Candeptin. Candicidin, *q.v.*

candicidin. An antifungal antibiotic, mainly used in vaginal candidiasis as vaginal tablets and ointment.

Canestan. Clotrimazole, *q.v.*

Capoten. Captopril, *q.v.*

capreomycin. An antibiotic of value in resistant tuberculosis or when other antibiotics are not tolerated. May cause deafness, tinnitus, renal damage and allergic reactions. Dose 1g daily by i.m. injection.

captopril. An inhibitor of the renin-angiotensin-enzyme system concerned with blood-pressure control. Used in severe hypertension resistant to standard therapy. Dose 25 to 150mg three times a day with food. May be used with thiazide diuretics, but treatment requires care and regular white cell counts. A pruritic skin rash may occur early.

carbachol. A parasympathomimetic agent used orally and by injection in the treatment of postoperative atony and retention of urine, and occasionally as eye drops in the treatment of glaucoma. Dose 2 to 4mg orally, 0.25 to 0.5mg by subcutaneous injection.

carbamazepine. An anticonvulsant effective in psychomotor epilepsy and grand mal, often in association with other drugs. Also effective in trigeminal neuralgia. Care is necessary in hepatic disease and glaucoma. Dose in epilepsy 200 to 1200mg daily, in neuralgia 100mg or more.

carbaryl. An insecticide used as a lotion and shampoo in pediculosis.

carbenicillin. A derivative of penicillin of lower potency but a wider range of activity. Of great value in systemic and urinary infections due to *Pseudomonas aeruginosa*, *Proteus*, and mixed infections. In severe systemic infections, large doses of 20 to 30g daily by rapid intravenous infusion are given; for urinary infections, 1 to 2g six-hourly by intramuscular injection. Smaller doses should be given when renal function is impaired.

carbenoxolone. A derivative of a compound obtained from liquorice. It has some anti-inflammatory properties resembling those of cortisone. Used in the ambulant treatment of gastric and duodenal ulcer, and locally for mouth ulcers. Side-effects include oedema and heartburn, and potassium supplements should be given to prevent hypokalaemia. Care is necessary in hepatic and renal dysfunction. Dose 150mg daily.

carbidopa. An enzyme inhibitor used with levodopa, *q.v.*, in parkinsonism. It prevents the breakdown of levodopa, thus permitting a larger amount to reach the brain.

carbimazole. An antithyroid drug. It inhibits the formation of thyroxine, *q.v.*, in the thyroid gland and is valuable for the oral treatment of thyrotoxicosis. May cause gastric disturbance in the early stages of treatment, but the drug may also cause fever and occasionally aplastic anaemia. Initial doses 30 to 60mg daily; maintenance doses 5 to 20mg daily.

carbocisteine. A mucolytic agent used to reduce the production and viscosity of sputum in respiratory disorders. Dose 750mg three times a day.

carbolic acid. Phenol, *q.v.*

carbon dioxide. A colourless, non-inflammable gas. It has a stimulating effect on the respiratory centre, and a mixture of 5% of carbon dioxide in oxygen is used for respiratory depression. Solid carbon dioxide is used to destroy warts, naevi, etc.

Cardophylin. Aminophylline, *q.v.*

carfecillin. An orally active

derivative that is broken down in the body to form carbenicillin, *q.v.* Used in urinary infections due to *Pseudomonas* and some other organisms. Not suitable for systemic infections. Dose 0.5 to 1g three times a day.

Carisoma. Carisprodol, *q.v.*

carisprodol. A muscle relaxant similar to mephenesin, *q.v.* Dose 350mg four times a day.

carmustine. A cytotoxic agent similar to lomustine, *q.v.*, but given by intravenous injection. Dose 100 to 250mg per square metre of body surface daily for two to three days. Delayed bone marrow depression is a dose-limiting factor.

Carylderm. Carbaryl, *q.v.*

cascara. A mild purgative. Dose: dry extract 100 to 250mg, liquid extract and elixir, 2 to 5ml.

castor oil. A mild purgative, often useful after food poisoning. Dose 5 to 20ml. The oil has emollient properties, and is used together with zinc ointment for pressure sores, and napkin rash.

Catapres. Clonidine, *q.v.*

catechu. A plant extract used with chalk, *q.v.*, in the treatment of diarrhoea. Dose of tincture of catechu 2 to 4ml.

Cedilanid. Lanatoside C, *q.v.*, and deslanoside C, *q.v.*

Cedocard. Isorbide dinitrate, *q.v.*

cefaclor. A cephalosporin, *q.v.*, type of antibiotic, used mainly in urinary and respiratory infections. Dose 250mg or more eight-hourly, up to a maximum of 2g.

cefamandole. A cephalosporin antibiotic more resistant to inactivation by penicillinases. Of value in serious infections resistant to other drugs. Dose 0.5 to 2g four- to six-hourly by injection.

cefotaxime. A cephalosporin, *q.v.*, type of antibiotic. Dose in urinary tract infections 1g i.m. or i.v. 12-hourly. For gonorrhoea, a single dose of 1g.

cefoxitin. A cephamycin antibiotic that is more resistant to beta-lactamase-producing Gram-negative organisms. It is useful in a wide range of infections resistant to some other antibiotics, and in peritonitis, but it is not active against *Pseudomonas* or *Enterococci*. Dose 1 to 2g eight-hourly by i.m. or i.v. injection. Care is necessary in hypersensitivity to cephalosporins, and in renal insufficiency.

cefuroxime. A cephalosporin type of antibiotic, often effective against some organisms resistant to penicillin. Dose up to 2g daily by i.m. or i.v. injection.

Celbenin. Methicillin, *q.v.*

Centrax. Prazepam, *q.v.*

cephalexin. An antibiotic similar in action and uses to cephaloridine, *q.v.*, but active orally. Used mainly in respiratory and urinary tract infections. May cause nausea and diarrhoea. Dose 250 to 500mg six-hourly.

cephaloridine. A bactericidal antibiotic effective against a wide range of organisms, including penicillin-resistant staphylococci, but not *Pseudomonas*. Of value in respiratory and urinary tract infections. Care is necessary in patients sensitive to penicillin, as cross-reactions of an allergic type may occur. Dose 0.5 to 1.5g by i.m. injection two or three times a day.

cephalosporins. A group of antibiotics related to the penicillins, but with a wider range of activity. Some are excreted unchanged, and are of value in urinary infections. See cephaloridine.

cephalothin. An antibiotic similar in action, uses and dose to cephaloridine, *q.v.* Often preferred if renal damage or dysfunction is present.

cephamycins. A small group of antibiotics closely related to the cephalosporins. See cefoxitin.

cephazolin. An antibiotic with the general properties of the cephaloridines. Given by i.m. injection in doses up to 2g daily in respiratory and genito-urinary infections.

cephradine. An orally active antibiotic similar in action and dose to cephalexin, *q.v.*

Ceporex. Cephalexin, *q.v.*

Ceporin. Cephaloridine, *q.v.*

Cetiprin. Emepronium, *q.v.*

cetrimide. A detergent with antiseptic properties, used chiefly in association with chlorhexidine, *q.v.*

chalk (calcium carbonate). An antacid used in treatment of peptic ulcer. Also given with astringents such as catechu in the treatment of diarrhoea. Dose 1 to 4g.

charcoal. A powerful adsorbent, given orally in flatulence, and to mark the passage of faeces. Large doses may be given as a first-aid measure in poisoning by many toxic substances. Dose 4 to 8g.

Chendol. Chenodeoxycholic acid, *q.v.*

chenodeoxycholic acid. This bile acid derivative has a solvent effect on cholesterol gallstones, and is useful when surgical removal of the stones is contra-indicated. It is given orally in doses of 1g daily, but prolonged treatment is required. Diarrhoea may limit treatment, and ursodeoxycholic acid, *q.v.*, is often preferred.

chloral hydrate. A water-soluble hypnotic with a prompt action. Of value for children and elderly patients. The drug must be given well diluted to reduce the gastric irritant effects. Dose 0.3 to 2g.

chlorambucil. An orally active cytostatic drug used in the treatment of malignant lymphoma and chronic lymphocytic leukaemia. It is relatively well tolerated, but strict haematological control of therapy is essential. Dose 5 to 10mg initially; 2 to 4mg daily.

chloramphenicol. An orally active antibiotic with a wide range of activity. Now used mainly in typhoid and para-typhoid fevers as damage to the blood-forming system may occur. Although effective in intestinal and urinary infections, in whooping cough, and in many rickettsial and viral infections, for these purposes less toxic drugs are now used. Chloramphenicol is also useful in skin and eye infections, and in otitis media. Average adult dose 500mg four times

a day, increased in severe infections. Children's doses range from 25 to 30mg per kg body-weight daily; but the drug may be dangerous for infants.

chlordiazepoxide. A psycho-therapeutic drug with tranquillising and muscle relaxant properties. Widely used in treatment of anxiety, tension, depression accompanied by agitation, and in alcoholism. Also useful in spastic neuro-muscular disorders. The drug has a wide margin of safety, and serious toxic effects are rare, but drowsiness and confusion may occur. Has been used by injection as a relaxant in tetanus. Dose 5 to 25mg orally, 50 to 100mg by injection.

chlorhexidine. An antiseptic of high potency and a wide range of activity, although it is ineffective against spores and viruses. It is well tolerated by the tissues. For skin preparation a 0.5% solution in methylated spirit is used, but for general use a mixture of chlorhexidine with cetrimide (Savlon) is often preferred. A general-purpose cream and an obstetric cream are also available. Solutions of chlorhexidine and other antiseptics may become contaminated with *Pseudomonas,* and all solutions should be freshly prepared and sterilised.

chlormethiazole. A sedative with anticonvulsant properties. Used by slow intravenous injection in acute mania, status epilepticus and toxaemia of pregnancy, and orally in alcoholism, epilepsy and insomnia. Oral dose 2 to 6g daily.

chlormezanone. A minor tranquilliser similar to meprobamate, *q.v.*, with some muscle relaxant action. Dose 200mg three or four times a day.

chlorocresol. A bactericide for injections in multiple-dose containers and in eye-drops.

chloroform. Once widely used as a general anaesthetic, but now obsolete. Used as chloroform water in mixtures as a preservative and flavouring agent, and for its carminative effects.

Chloromycetin. Chloramphenicol, *q.v.*

chloroquine. An anti-malarial drug effective against the erythrocytic forms of malarial parasites and used both for the suppression and treatment of malaria. Suppressive dose 0.3g weekly. Treatment 0.6g initially, followed by 0.3g six to eight hours later, then 0.3g daily for two days.

chlorothiazide. The first of the widely used group of thiazide diuretics. These drugs have a marked salt and water-eliminating action and are highly effective and well tolerated. Occasional side-effects include allergy, nausea and, rarely, some blood disorders. Chlorothiazide and related compounds are used extensively in congestive heart failure, and oedematous states generally. They are also used in hypertension, as they increase the activity of many antihypertensive agents and permit lower doses and reduce associated side-effects. Some potassium as well as sodium loss is caused by these drugs, and potassium chloride should be given to offset such loss if treatment is prolonged. Dose of chlorothiazide 0.5 to 2g daily. Newer derivatives are effective in much lower doses.

chlorotrianisene. A synthetic oestrogen which after absorption is taken up by the body fat, from which it is slowly released to give a prolonged action. Used in menopausal conditions; for the suppression of lactation, and in prostatic carcinoma. Side-effects such as nausea are uncommon. Dose 12 to 48mg daily.

chloroxylenol. A non-irritating

germicide, widely used in many non-caustic antiseptics. Although effective against streptococci, it is less active against staphylococci, and of no value against *Ps. aeruginosa* or *Proteus*.

chlorpheniramine. A potent antihistamine with few side-effects. Active orally in doses of 4 to 16mg daily. Also of value in the treatment of transfusion reactions and doses of 10mg may be added to an intravenous drip solution.

chlorpromazine. A major tranquilliser with a wide range of activity on the central nervous system. It is widely employed as an anti-emetic; for potentiating the action of analgesics and hypnotics; for its powerful tranquillising action in the treatment of agitation, tension and other psychiatric conditions; and the management of refractory and schizophrenic patients. Oral dose 25 to 50mg, increased in mental disorders. Similar doses may be given by intravenous or deep intramuscular injection. It should not be given subcutaneously. It may cause obstructive jaundice in some patients, and blood dyscrasia may also occur. Care should be taken in handling any solution of the drug, as skin

sensitisation may occur after contact.

chlorpropamide. An oral hypoglycaemic agent of the sulphonylurea type, and acts by stimulating the production and release of insulin. It is effective only if the insulin-secreting cells are still functional. It is used mainly in the treatment of mild diabetes mellitus occurring in middle-aged patients. The drug is sometimes effective in patients who do not respond to tolbutamide, *q.v.*, and in other cases may permit the insulin requirements to be reduced. Side-effects include rash, jaundice and blood dyscrasia, but are uncommon with low doses. Dose 250 to 500mg daily as a single morning dose.

chlorprothixene. A tranquilliser related chemically to chlorpromazine, *q.v.* It is used for similar purposes and has similar side-effects. Of value in acute conditions, less suitable for maintenance therapy. Dose 30 to 600mg daily.

chlortetracycline. An orally effective antibiotic with the general properties of tetracyclines, *q.v.* Chlortetracycline may be given intravenously in emergency, but solutions must be injected very slowly, as vein inflammation may occur. Dose: oral, 250 to 500mg six-hourly.

chlorthalidone. A diuretic similar in action and uses to hydrochlorothiazide, *q.v.* Dose 100 to 200mg daily.

Choledyl. A derivative of theophylline, *q.v.*, with reduced gastric irritant effects.

cholestyramine. An exchange resin that binds bile salts in the intestines, so that they are excreted in the faeces. It is used in some forms of hyperlipoproteinaemia, and to relieve the pruritus associated with biliary obstruction. Dose 10 to 16g daily.

chorionic gonadotrophin. A gonad-stimulating hormone derived from the placenta. It has been used in anovulatory sterility, metropathia haemorrhagica, habitual abortion, and undescended testicle. Dose 500 to 1000 units by intramuscular injection.

chymotrypsin. A proteolytic enzyme of the pancreas. Used to reduce soft tissue oedema and inflammation. Dose 20 000 units or more orally four times a day, or 5000 units by i.m. injection. Also used in ophthalmology to facilitate intracapsular lens extraction.

Ciba 1906. Thiambutosine, *q.v.*

ciclacillin. A broad spectrum penicillin type antibiotic. Dose 250 to 500mg six-hourly. In cases of renal inefficiency, the dosage interval should be extended.

Cidex. Glutaraldehyde, *q.v.*

Cidomycin. Gentamicin, *q.v.*

cimetidine. A powerful histamine H_2 receptor antagonist. Unlike ordinary antihistamines, it inhibits gastric secretion, and is used in the treatment of peptic ulcer and other conditions of gastric hyperacidity. Dose 200mg three times a day, and 400mg at night. May cause diarrhoea and other side-effects.

cinchocaine. A local anaesthetic of high potency. Ointment, cream and suppositories are available.

cinnarizine. An antihistamine chiefly of value in Ménière's disease and motion sickness. Dose 45 to 90mg daily.

Cinobac. Cinoxacin, *q.v.*

Cinoxacin. An antibacterial agent with actions, uses and side-effects similar to nalidixic acid, *q.v.* Dose 500mg twice a day.

cisplatin. An unusual cytotoxic agent that contains platinum as an organic complex. Used in metastatic ovarian and testicular tumours, and in refractory malignant disease. Dose 10 to 20mg per square metre body surface intravenously daily, for five days a month according to need. Toxic effects include nausea, deafness and renal damage.

Citanest. Prilocaine, *q.v.*

Claforan. Cefotaxime, *q.v.*

clemastine. An antihistamine used in allergic rhinitis, urticaria and allergic dermatoses. Dose 1mg twice a day, up to a maximum of 6mg daily.

clindamycin. An antibiotic with actions and uses similar to lincomycin, *q.v.* Dose 150 to 450mg six-hourly.

Clinium. Lidoflazine, *q.v.*

Clinoril. Sulindac, *q.v.*

clobazam. A benzodiazepine tranquilliser with the actions and uses of diazepam, *q.v.* Said to have reduced psychomotor side-effects. Dose 30 to 60mg daily, reduced as required.

clobetasol. A potent locally acting corticosteroid used in a wide variety of inflamed skin conditions. Care is necessary, as absorption with systemic effects on the pituitary-adrenal system may occur if treatment is prolonged.

clobetasone. A locally acting corticosteroid of value in the milder forms of eczema and other steroid-responsive conditions. Of particular value in young children, who

may be more sensitive to the undesirable effects of local steroids.

clofazimine. An antileprotic agent, of value in conditions resistant to dapsone, *q.v.* May cause discolouration of the skin and lesions. Dose 200 to 600mg weekly.

clofibrate. A drug which lowers the level of cholesterol and triglycerides in the blood, and so of value in atherosclerosis. May potentiate the action of anticoagulants, the dose of which should be reduced during clofibrate treatment. Not advised during pregnancy. Dose 1.5 to 2g daily.

Clomid. Clomiphene, *q.v.*

clomiphene. Has some oestrogen-like properties, and is used in anovulatory sterility. Dose 50mg daily for 5 days a month, repeated if ovulation does not occur. If pregnancy does not follow up to six courses, further treatment is of little use. Contra-indicated in hepatic disease and ovarian neoplasm.

clomipramine. A tricyclic antidepressant with an action basically similar to that of imipramine, *q.v.* It has the side-effects of anticholinergic drugs. Dose 30 to 150mg daily.

clomocycline. A derivative of tetracycline, with a similar range of anti-bacterial activity; but absorbed and excreted more rapidly, and effective in the lower dose of 170mg six-hourly.

clonazepam. A drug related to diazepam, *q.v.*, but it has marked anticonvulsant properties. Used in all types of epilepsy in doses adjusted to age and response. Often causes drowsiness. Adult dose from 4 to 8mg daily. In status epilepticus, 1mg intravenously.

clonidine. A potent antihypertensive agent, effective in small doses, and often of value when guanethidine is not tolerated. Dose 75 micrograms initially, increased slowly to a daily dose of 1mg or more. In doses of 50 micrograms daily, it is used in the prophylactic treatment of migraine.

clopamide. A diuretic with an action similar to chlorothiazide, but with a more rapid and reliable effect. Dose 20 to 60mg daily, or as necessary, taken at morning to avoid nocturia. As with other diuretics some potassium loss may occur. Clopamide also has some antihypertensive properties.

clopenthixol. A powerful tranquilliser with the actions, uses and side-effects of chlorpromazine, *q.v.* Used

mainly in schizophrenia with agitation. Dose 200mg to 400mg by intramuscular injection every two to four weeks.

Clopixol. Clopenthixol, *q.v.*

clorazepate. A benzodiazepine tranquilliser with the actions and uses of diazepam, *q.v.* Used mainly in the treatment of anxiety with a single nightly dose of 15mg; but larger, divided doses are sometimes required.

clorexolone. A diuretic with the action, uses and side-effects of chlorothiazide, but effective in lower doses which have a longer action. Dose 25 to 100mg daily or alternate days.

clotrimazole. An antimycotic for vaginal infections. Used as vaginal tablets, 200mg for insertion nightly; also as vaginal cream.

cloxacillin. A semi-synthetic penicillin that is not broken down by the enzyme penicillinase, and so is effective against resistant staphylococci. Oral adult dose is 500mg six-hourly; in severe infections given by injection in doses of 250 to 500mg six-hourly. Now largely replaced by flucloxacillin, *q.v.* The side-effects are those of the penicillins generally.

coal tar. The black viscous

liquid obtained from the distillation of coal. It is used mainly as Zinc and Tar Paste in eczema, psoriasis and pruritus.

cocaine. A powerful local anaesthetic. Now largely replaced by less toxic compounds. Still used occasionally in ophthalmology as a 2% solution, often with homatropine, *q.v.*

cod-liver oil. A rich source of vitamins A and D. It is used as a dietary supplement to improve general nutrition, promote calcification and prevent rickets. Dose 2 to 10ml daily.

codeine. One of the alkaloids of opium. It depresses the cough centre and is widely prescribed for the treatment of useless cough. It also has mild analgesic properties, and is used with aspirin in Compound Codeine Tablets and similar preparations. In large doses the constipating action of codeine may be a disadvantage. Dose 10 to 60mg.

Cogentin. Benztropine, *q.v.*

colaspase. An enzyme that breaks down the amino-acid asparagine, which is essential for the development of some malignant cells. Colaspase thus has an indirect effect on the growth of such cells. Used mainly in acute leukaemia.

Dose 200 units per kg body-weight daily by slow intravenous injection.

colchicine. The alkaloid obtained from the meadow saffron. It is used in acute gout, and is given in doses of 0.5mg every two hours until relief is obtained. A total dose of 6mg should not be exceeded, but relief of pain or the onset of vomiting or diarrhoea usually renders full doses unnecessary.

Colestid. Colestipol, *q.v.*

colestipol. An exchange resin that binds bile salts in the gut, and so prevents reabsorption, and indirectly reduces the synthesis of cholesterol. Used in hypercholesterolaemia in doses of 15 to 30g daily. May interfere with the absorption of many drugs.

colistin. An antibiotic chiefly effective against Gram-negative organisms, and given orally in gastro-enteritis. For systemic and urinary infections it must be given by injection in doses of 2 mega units eight-hourly. Less toxic antibiotics are now usually preferred. Side-effects after injection include neurotoxic and nephrotoxic symptoms.

collodion. A solution of pyroxylin used as a protective dressing to small wounds.

Colofac. Mebeverine, *q.v.*

Colomycin. Colistin, *q.v.*

Concordin. Protriptyline, *q.v.*

congo red. A red dye used by intravenous injection as a 1% solution in the diagnosis of amyloid disease. The degree of absorption of the dye from the blood one hour after injection is measured, and a loss of more than 30% is an indication of amyloid disease.

Coparvax. A preparation of inactivated *Corynebacterium parvum* organisms. It is used by injection into the pleural or peritoneal cavity (after aspiration) in the treatment of malignant pleural effusion and malignant ascites. Dose 7 to 14mg, repeated if necessary after 7 days.

copper sulphate. The main constituent of Clinitest tablets and Benedict's solution used for testing for glucose in urine.

Coptin. Co-trimazine, *q.v.*

Cordarone X. Amiodarone, *q.v.*

Cordilox. Verapamil, *q.v.*

Corgard. Nadolol, *q.v.*

Corlan. A hydrocortisone preparation for mouth ulcers.

corticotrophin. The adreno-corticotrophic hormone of the anterior pituitary gland. It stimulates the production of corticoid hormones by the adrenal cortex, especially hydrocortisone, and hence has a wide range of activity. The drug has a rapid action and is very useful in the treatment of severe asthma and allergic states and in some inflammatory conditions. It is not effective in adrenal deficiency states, where replacement therapy with cortisone is necessary. The dose varies from 10 to 25 units four times a day by intramuscular or subcutaneous injection, but long-acting forms are also avilable. The effects are often dramatic but slow withdrawal of treatment is essential. The side-effects are due to pituitary imbalance, and may include Cushing's syndrome, water and salt retention, and mental disturbances. Contra-indicated in peptic ulcer, hypertension and tuberculosis. Care is necessary in diabetes.

cortisone. One of the most important of the steroid hormones secreted by the adrenal cortex. Together with hydrocortisone, it plays a major part in the body metabolism, controlling the formation of glucose, the salt and water balance, the resistance to stress, and the response to inflammatory and allergic stimuli. Side-effects include hypertension and oedema due to disturbance of the electrolyte balance, and retention of salt and water, mental disturbances, reactivation of peptic ulcer, and increased liability to infection. Cortisone is used mainly in Addison's disease and related conditions, where its salt-retaining action is an advantage. In other systemic conditions, such as rheumatoid arthritis, leukaemia and other blood disorders, and for immunosuppresion in transplant surgery, this salt-retaining action is undesirable, and many alternative drugs such as prednisone, *q.v.*, triamcinolone and betamethasone have a more specific action. Dose of cortisone 50 to 400mg daily, orally, or by i.m. injection, based upon need and response, later slowly reduced and eventually withdrawn.

co-trimazine. Trimethaprim, *q.v.*, and sulphadiazine, *q.v.*

co-trimoxazole. A B.N.F. preparation containing sulphamethoxazole, *q.v.*, and trimethaprim, *q.v.* The combination has an increased antibacterial action.

Cosmegen. Actinomycin D, *q.v.*

Crasnitin. Colaspase, *q.v.*

cresol. A powerful antiseptic similar to phenol. It is the principal constituent of lysol, *q.v.*

crotamiton. An ascaricide and antipruritic. Used by local application as cream or lotion (10%) in the treatment of scabies and itching conditions.

crystal violet. A dyestuff with a selective antiseptic action against Gram-positive organisms and yeasts. Used as a 0.5% solution for burns and infected skin conditions. An alcoholic solution with brilliant green is used for skin preparation.

Cuprimine. Penicillamine, *q.v.*

cyanocobalamin. The antianaemic factor present in liver. It is specific in the treatment of pernicious anaemia, and its neurological complications, and of value in some other anaemias due to nutritional deficiencies. In large doses it has been used for the relief of certain neurological conditions such as herpes zoster. Dose in pernicious anaemia 1000 micrograms or more, once or twice weekly by i.m. injection. Maintenance doses of 250 micrograms at longer intervals. Cyanocobalamin is rapidly excreted, and for maintenance hydroxocobalamin, *q.v.*, is often preferred.

cyclandelate. A peripheral vasodilator used in circulatory disorders such as acrocyanosis and vasospasm. May be useful in cerebrovascular disease. Side-effects include nausea and dizziness. Dose 400 to 800mg or more daily.

cyclizine. An antihistamine used mainly in travel sickness and nausea generally. Also useful in vertigo. Dose 50mg two or three times a day.

cyclobarbitone. A short-acting barbiturate with the general sedative action of that group of drugs. Dose 200 to 400mg.

cyclopenthiazide. One of the thiazide group of diuretics. Effective in many oedematous conditions, and also in hypertension as an adjuvant to other antihypertensive drugs. Dose 1mg initially, 250 to 500 micrograms daily as necessary.

cyclopentolate. An anticholinergic agent used to produce cycloplegia and mydriasis. The action is more rapid and less prolonged than atropine.

cyclophosphamide. A cytostatic drug, active orally and by injection, with an action similar to mustine. Used in Hodgkin's disease and other cancerous conditions. Dose 100 to 150mg daily, orally or i.v.

cyclopropane. An inhalation anaesthetic of high potency with which induction and recovery are rapid. It causes some respiratory depression

and cardiac irregularities, and its administration requires care. It is used with closed-circuit apparatus. Supplied in orange-coloured cylinders.

cycloserine. An antibiotic active chiefly against the tubercle bacillus, and used in severe pulmonary tuberculosis when standard drugs are ineffective. Occasionally used in urinary infections. Dose 250 to 750mg daily.

Cyclospasmol. Cyclandelate, *q.v.*

cyclosporin A. A fungal metabolite that has unusual immunosuppressive properties. It is under investigation as an immunosuppressive agent in transplant surgery, but its true value has yet to be assessed.

Cyklokapron. Tranexamic acid, *q.v.*

cyproheptadine. A powerful antihistamine and antiserotonin compound. Some allergic reactions are due not only to histamine, but also to serotonin, and cyproheptadine is useful in conditions not responding completely to an antihistamine. Dose 4 to 20mg daily.

cyproterone. An anti-androgen used to reduce libido in sexual deviants. Dose 50 to 300mg daily. Care necessary in liver disease and diabetes.

Not effective in chronic alcoholics.

Cytamen. Cyanocobalamin, *q.v.*

cytarabine. A cytostatic agent that prevents cell development by inhibiting the formation of nucleic acid. May induce remission in acute leukaemia. Dose 3mg per kg body-weight daily by i.v. injection, according to response.

Cytosar. Cytarabine, *q.v.*

D

DDT. Dicophane, *q.v.*

DDVAP. Desmopressin, *q.v.*

DF118. Dihydrocodeine, *q.v.*

DMSO. Dimethyl sulphoxide, *q.v.*

DOCA. Deoxycortone acetate, *q.v.*

DTIC. Dacarbazine, *q.v.*

dacarbazine. A cytotoxic drug that appears to influence purine metabolism. Used in melanoma and Hodgkin's disease. Dose 2 to 4.5mg/kg i.v. daily for 10 days. Care in handling; skin irritant.

Dactil. Piperidolate, *q.v.*

Daktarin. Miconazole, *q.v.*

Dalacin C. Clindamycin, *q.v.*

Dalmane. Flurazepam, *q.v.*

danazol. A derivative of ethisterone that inhibits the release of pituitary gonadotrophins. Used in conditions such as endometriosis, gynaecomastia and precocious puberty. Care is necessary in cardiac, renal and hepatic dysfunction. Dose 100 to 800mg daily.

Danol. Danazol, *q.v.*

Dantrium. Dantrolene, *q.v.*

dantrolene. A skeletal muscle relaxant that appears to act within the muscle fibre, and not at the myoneural junction. Used in severe spastic states following stroke and spinal cord injury. Dose 25mg initially, increasing to 400mg daily as required. May cause hepatotoxicity, and its use needs care. An intravenous preparation is available for use in malignant hyperthermia. Dose 1mg/kg as soon as condition is diagnosed, repeated as necessary up to a total dose of 10mg/kg.

Daonil. Glibenclamide, *q.v.*

dapsone. A sulphone compound used in the treatment of lepromatous and tuberculoid leprosy and in dermatitis herpetiformis. Dose: orally, 25 to 100mg twice weekly in leprosy; daily doses of 50 to 200mg in dermatitis herpetiformis. Also used with pyrimethamine, *q.v.*, as Maloprim in chloroquine-resistant malaria.

Daranide. Dichlorphenamide, *q.v.*

Daraprim. Pyrimethamine, *q.v.*

Dartalan. Thiopropazate, *q.v.*

debrisoquine. A well-tolerated antihypertensive drug of the guanethidine type, effective in all types of hypertension, including those not responding to other drugs. Initial dose 20mg, increasing by 10mg to maintenance doses of 40 to 120mg daily. Side-effects may be reduced by combined treatment with a thiazide diuretic.

Decadron. Dexamethasone, *q.v.*

Decaserpyl. Methoserpidine, *q.v.*

Declinax. Debrisoquine, *q.v.*

demecarium. An enzyme inhibitor used like timolol, *q.v.*, in glaucoma. Eye drops 0.25% and 0.5%.

demeclocycline. A tetracycline antibiotic with a wide range of activity. Allergic and phototoxic reactions may be more frequent than with similar drugs. Has caused polyuria by blocking action of the anti-diuretic hormone. Dose 150mg six-hourly.

Dendrid. Idoxuridine, *q.v.*

deoxycortone. One of the hormones of the cortex of the adrenal gland, controlling sodium retention and potassium excretion. Occasionally used in the treatment of Addison's disease and to supplement cortisone

therapy. Dose 2 to 10mg by i.m. injection.

Depixol. Flupenthixol, *q.v.*

Depostat. Gestronol, *q.v.*

Depot-Provera. Medroxy-progesterone, *q.v.*

Derbac. Preparations of malathion, *q.v.*, and carbaryl, *q.v.*

Dermovate. Clobetasol, *q.v.*

Deseril. Methysergide, *q.v.*

deserpidine. A derivative of reserpine, *q.v.*

Desferal. Desferrioxamine, *q.v.*

desferrioxamine. A substance that combines with iron salts to form a soluble non-toxic complex. Of great value in acute iron poisoning in children. Dose 2g immediately by i.m. injection, together with 5g orally.

desipramine. A derivative of imipramine, *q.v.*, with similar antidepressant properties, but with a more rapid action. A response may be apparent within a week of treatment. Dose: 25 to 75mg, increasing to 200mg daily orally, 25 to 50mg by i.m. injection.

deslanoside C. A derivative of lanatoside C, *q.v.*, suitable for injection. Used for rapid digitalisation and in emergencies such as pulmonary oedema. Dose 0.8 to 1.2mg, i.v., reduced according to need.

desmopressin. A derivative of vasopressin, *q.v.*, with increased potency and longer duration of action. Used in the diagnosis and control of diabetes insipidus. Dose 10 to 20 micrograms intranasally; 1 to 4 micrograms daily by injection.

Destolit. Ursodeoxycholic acid, *q.v.*

dexamethasone. A synthetic corticosteroid with reduced salt-retaining properties. Useful in all conditions requiring glucocorticoid therapy except Addison's disease. Dose 0.5 to 10mg daily.

dexamphetamine sulphate. A central nervous system stimulant similar to amphetamine, *q.v.*; but it also has appetite-depressant properties. Dose 5 to 10mg.

Dexedrine. Dexamphetamine sulphate, *q.v.*

dextran. A blood-plasma substitute obtained from sucrose solutions by bacterial action. Of value in burns, shock, etc., when blood or plasma is not available. Special dextran solutions are used to reduce blood viscosity and red cell aggregation, and to improve peripheral circulation.

dextromoramide. A synthetic morphine-like analgesic of value in severe and intractable pain. Care is necessary in liver dysfunction and respiratory depression. Dose 5mg or more either orally or

by injection, according to need and response.

dextropropoxyphene. An orally effective analgesic present in Distalgesic. Of value in many painful conditions, and in malignant disease, its use may delay the need to resort to the opiate analgesics. Dose 30 to 60mg. Excessive doses may have toxic effects such as analgesic nephropathy.

dextrose. A readily absorbed carbohydrate found in many sweet fruits, but obtained commercially by the hydrolysis of starch. It is given orally as a dietary supplement; in acidosis; and to raise the glycogen reserve of the liver in poisoning by drugs causing hepatic damage. Given by i.v. injection as a 5% solution or as dextrose-saline in severe dehydration, shock, and after abdominal operations until fluids can again be taken orally.

Diaginol. Sodium acetrizoate, *q.v.*

Diabinese. Chlorpropamide, *q.v.*

diamorphine. A derivative of morphine with a more powerful analgesic and cough-suppressant action. Valuable for the relief of severe pain and the suppression of useless cough. Addiction is a constant risk owing to the euphoric effects of the drug, and the use of diamorphine, except in terminal cases, has declined as more satisfactory morphine-like analgesics have become available. Dose 5 to 10mg or more as required.

Diamox. Acetazolamide, *q.v.*

Dianabol. Methandienone, *q.v.*

diazepam. A tranquillising drug similar to chlordiazepoxide, *q.v.*, and of value in anxiety states. It is useful for premedication as well as psychiatric states. It has a muscle relaxant action, and is valuable when given by injection in status asthmaticus, and in the control of the spasm of tetanus. Dose 5 to 30mg daily, 2 to 10mg by injection as required, up to a maximum of 30mg in eight hours.

diazoxide. An inhibitor of insulin secretion. Used intravenously in severe hypoglycaemia in doses of 2 to 5mg per kg body-weight. Also of value in severe hypertensive crisis in doses of 300mg by rapid intravenous injection.

Dibenyline. Phenoxybenzamine, *q.v.*

Dibotin. Phenformin, *q.v.*

dichloralphenazone. A combination of chloral and phenazone. The product is better tolerated than chloral, and causes less gastric disturbance. It is given as tablets of 650mg, equivalent to 400mg of chloral hydrate.

dichlorphenamide. An inhibitor of carbonic anhydrase. Used in glaucoma, and in the chronic respiratory insufficiency of acute bronchitis. Dose 25 to 50mg. Long-term treatment may cause electrolyte disturbance.

diclofenac. One of many non-steroidal anti-inflammatory agents such as fenbufen or naproxen. Dose 25 to 50mg three times a day after meals. Suppositories 100mg useful at night.

Diconal. Dipipanone, *q.v.*

dicophane (DDT). An effective but slow-acting contact insecticide; valuable in the elimination of body parasites as dicophane application (2%), or dusting powder (10%).

dicyclomine. A synthetic atropine-like compound, used to reduce hyperacidity and for its antispasmodic action in peptic ulcer, biliary spasm, colic and pylorospasm. Dose 10 to 20mg.

Dicynene. Ethamsylate, *q.v.*

Didronal. Disodium etidronate, *q.v.*

dienoestrol. Synthetic oestrogen similar to stilboestrol, *q.v.* Dose 1 to 10mg.

diethylcarbamazine. A synthetic drug used in filariasis. Effective chiefly against microfilariae, and thus reduces spread of the disease by insects. Longer treatment is necessary to kill the adult worms. Dose 150 to 500mg daily. Low initial doses may be necessary to reduce allergic reactions due to proteins released from dead worms.

diethylpropion. An appetite depressant related chemically to the amphetamines, but with reduced central stimulant effects. Dose 25mg.

diflucortolone. A corticosteroid used topically as a 0.1% or 0.3% cream or ointment in steroid-responsive dermatoses. Of value in resistant conditions.

diflunisal. An anti-inflammatory and analgesic drug related to aspirin, but less liable to cause gastro-intestinal disturbances. Useful in arthritic and other conditions where a prolonged action is required. Dose 250mg twice a day. Care is necessary in aspirin-sensitive patients, or in peptic ulcer.

Digitaline Nativelle. Preparations of digitoxin, *q.v.* Tablets or granules of 0.1mg and 0.25mg, oral solution 1:1000, ampoules 0.2mg for i.m. injection.

digitalis. The leaf of the foxglove. It has a powerful strengthening and regula-

tory action on the heart, but is now used mainly as digoxin, *q.v.*

digitoxin. The most powerful cardiac glycoside of digitalis leaf. Absorption is rapid but excretion is very slow, and cumulative effects may occur. Maintenance dose, which requires careful adjustment, varies from 50 to 200 micrograms daily, but larger doses may be given initially.

digoxin. A powerful cardiac glycoside obtained from digitalis leaf. It is rapidly absorbed orally, and is widely used in cardiac failure, as it has a stimulant effect on the myocardium. Also of value in paroxysmal tachycardia and atrial fibrillation. The diuresis of digoxin therapy is a secondary effect following on the improvement in the renal circulation. Dose for rapid digitalisation 1 to 1.5mg initially; subsequent maintenance dose 0.25mg once or twice daily. For slow digitalisation, 0.5 to 1mg may be given daily for about a week, with subsequent doses based on the response. Elderly patients and children respond adequately to smaller doses, and tablets of 0.0625mg are available. In emergency, digoxin can be given by i.m. or slow i.v.

injection. Nausea and vomiting are often signs of overdose, and a dose should be omitted if the heart rate falls below 60 beats per minute.

Dihydergot. Dihydroergotamine, *q.v.*

dihydrocodeine. An analgesic derived from codeine, but with a more powerful action. Of value in many painful conditions where mild analgesics are inadequate. Dose 30 to 60mg orally or by injection.

dihydroergotamine. A derivative of ergotamine, *q.v.*, but with reduced pressor effects. It can be used in the prophylaxis as well as the treatment of migraine. Dose 1 to 2mg three times a day for prophylaxis; 2 to 3mg half-hourly, as necessary, up to a total dose of 10mg for treatment. May also be given by injection in doses of 1 to 2mg. Usually well tolerated.

dihydrotachysterol. A sterol related to calciferol, *q.v.*, but with more rapid calcium-mobilising properties. It is used mainly in hypocalcaemia and parathyroid tetany, but is sometimes effective in calciferol-resistant rickets. Given as an oily solution (AT 10, *q.v.*) in doses of 0.5ml or more according to the blood-calcium level. The therapeutic dose is often close to the toxic dose that may cause kidney calcification.

diloxanide. An amoebicide used only in intestinal amoebiasis. Dose 1.5g daily for 10 days.

Dimelor. Acetohexamide, *q.v.*

dimenhydrinate. An anti-emetic drug similar to some antihistamines. Used mainly to prevent travel sickness, vomiting of pregnancy, and radiation sickness. Dose 50mg.

dimercaprol. (BAL). A clear liquid, used in the treatment of poisoning by arsenic, mercury and gold. Given by i.m. injection as 5% solution in arachis oil. Dose 8 to 16ml in divided doses for one day, subsequent doses of 2 to 4ml daily according to need.

dimethicone. Activated dimethicone is an anti-foaming agent, said to reduce flatulence and protect mucous membranes. It is a constituent of many antacid preparations.

dimethyl sulphoxide. A solvent which penetrates the skin to an unusual degree. It has some anti-inflammatory properties, but is used mainly as a solvent for idoxuridine, *q.v.*, for use in cutaneous herpes.

Dimotane. Brompheniramine, *q.v.*

Dindevan. Phenindione, *q.v.*

dinoprostone. A synthetic form of prostaglandin E_2. It initiates contractions of the pregnant uterus, and has been used orally and intravenously in doses of 0.5mg to initiate labour. Larger doses have been given to terminate pregnancy. Its availability is restricted to approved centres.

dioctyl sodium sulphosuccinate. Docusate, *q.v.*

diodone injection. A solution of a complex organic iodine compound, used as a contrast agent in x-ray examination of kidneys and ureters. Stronger solutions are used in angiocardiography, etc. Dose 20ml i.v.

diphenhydramine. One of the early antihistamines. Used in the treatment of allergic conditions, including urticaria, rhinitis, atopic dermatitis, hay fever, and drug reactions. It also has a sedative action, which in some allergic conditions is an advantage. Also useful in travel sickness. Dose 50 to 200mg daily.

diphenoxylate. A derivative of pethidine which has no analgesic properties, but reduces intestinal activity. Used as Lomotil, *q.v.*, in the treatment of diarrhoea. Lomotil contains a small dose of atropine, to prevent abuse, as excessive doses of diphenoxylate may produce a morphine-like dependence.

diphenylpyraline. An antihistamine similar to promethazine, *q.v.*, but with reduced sedative effects. Dose 5 to 20mg daily.

dipipanone. A rapidly-acting and powerful analgesic similar to methadone, *q.v.* Usually given orally with cyclizine as Diconal. Dose 10 to 30mg six-hourly. May be given by intramuscular injection (intravenous use causes a marked fall in blood pressure).

Dipidolor. Piritramide, *q.v.*

dipyridamole. A coronary vasodilator used in the prophylaxis of chronic angina. Of no value in acute angina. May reduce platelet aggregation in cardiovascular disease. Dose 50 to 100mg three times a day.

Disalcid. Salsalate, *q.v.*

Disipal. Orphenadrine, *q.v.*

Di-Sipidin. Pituitary extract in powder form for use as a snuff in diabetes insipidus and enuresis. Careful application of the snuff is essential to obtain the maximum effects

disodium edetate. Sodium edetate, *q.v.*

disodium etidronate. A diphosphonate that inhibits excessive bone demineralisation.

Of value in Paget's disease, and in reducing the risk of fractures. Dose 5mg/kg as a single daily dose for up to six months. Care is necessary in renal impairment.

disopyramide. A quinidine-like drug used in the oral treatment of cardiac arrhythmias. The dose varies from 300 to 800mg daily according to need. Care is necessary if a degree of heart block is present, and by its anticholinergic action, glaucoma and urinary retention are contra-indications.

Distaclor. Cefaclor, *q.v.*

Distalgesic. See dextropropoxyphene.

Distamine. Penicillamine, *q.v.*

distigmine. An inhibitor of cholinesterase similar to neostigmine, *q.v.,* used orally mainly in the treatment of neurogenic bladder, and by injection in postoperative urinary retention. Dose 5mg orally, 500 micrograms by i.m. injection.

disulfiram. Tetraethylthiuram disulphide. When taken in association with alcohol, side-effects such as flushing, giddiness, vomiting and headache occur and may be severe. Acute confusion may occur if given at the same time as metronidazole. The drug has been used in chronic alcoholism, but pro-longed treatment and co-operation of the patient are essential. Dose 200 to 400mg daily.

dithranol. Synthetic compound used mainly in the treatment of psoriasis. The drug is a powerful irritant, and treatment should be commenced with a simple ointment or zinc paste containing 0.1%, gradually increased to 1% if well tolerated.

Diurexan. Xipamide, *q.v.*

Dixarit. Clonidine, *q.v.*, for the prophylactic treatment of migraine.

dobutamine. A sympathomimetic agent similar to isoprenaline, *q.v.,* but with a more selective action on the B_1 receptors in the heart, and less likely to cause tachycardia. Useful in acute heart failure and shock. Given by i.v. infusion in doses of 2.5 to 10 microgram/kg/minute, carefully adjusted to need.

Dobutrex. Dobutamine, *q.v.*

docusate. A surface-active agent used as a faeces-softening laxative.

Dolobid. Diflunisal, *q.v.*

Doloxene. Dextropropoxyphene, *q.v.*

domiphen bromide. A detergent antiseptic similar to cetrimide, *q.v.* Lozenges for throat infections are available.

domperidone. A new type of

anti-emetic that does not cause sedation or other central side-effects. Effective in acute nausea and vomiting, including that following cancer chemotherapy or irradiation. Dose 10 to 20mg orally or by injection.

dopamine. A sympathomimetic agent related to noradrenaline, *q.v.*, but with a more selective dilator action on renal and mesenteric blood vessels. Used mainly in shock by slow intravenous infusion in carefully controlled doses of 2 to 5 microgram/kg/ minute. In larger doses it also increases cardiac output. In parkinsonism, normal brain levels of dopamine are reduced, but the loss can be restored by levodopa, *q.v.*

Dopram. Doxapram, *q.v.*

Doriden. Glutethimide, *q.v.*

dothiepin. A tricyclic antidepressant with the uses and side-effects of imipramine, *q.v.* Dose 75 to 150mg daily.

doxapram. A respiratory stimulant useful in postoperative respiratory depression, or that caused by narcotic analgesics. Dose, by intravenous infusion, 0.5 to 4mg per minute.

doxepin. An antidepressant of the imipramine type, but with additional tranquillising properties. Used in the treatment of depression accompanied by anxiety. Dose 30 to 300mg daily.

doxorubicin. An antibiotic with cytostatic properties. Used in leukaemia and lymphosarcoma. Toxic effects may limit treatment. Dose 0.5mg per kg body-weight daily by intravenous injection.

doxycycline. A long-acting tetracycline derivative. Following an initial dose of 200mg an adequate antibacterial blood leven can be maintained by a single daily dose of 100mg.

Dramamine. Dimenhydrinate, *q.v.*

Droleptan. Droperidol, *q.v.*

Dromoran. Levorphanol, *q.v.*

droperidol. A tranquilliser with unusual properties. Used mainly with analgesics to produce a state of detachment before various diagnostic procedures.

drostanolone. A synthetic steroid with some of the anabolic and androgenic properties of testosterone. Of value in the treatment of carcinoma of the breast in doses of 100mg once to three times a week by i.m. injection.

Dryptal. Frusemide, *q.v.*

Dulcolax. Bisacodyl, *q.v.*

Duogastrone. Carbenoxolone, *q.v.*, in a capsule for the treatment of duodenal ulcer.

Duphalac. Lactulose, *q.v.*

Duphaston. Dydrogesterone, *q.v.*

Durabolin. Nandrolone, *q.v.*

Durophet. A long-acting product containing amphetamine, *q.v.* Used as an appetite depressant in obesity.

Duvalidan. Isoxuprine, *q.v.*

dydrogesterone. An orally active progestogen that is virtually free from any oestrogenic or androgenic side-effects. It does not inhibit ovulation, and is used in amenorrhoea, functional uterine bleeding, and threatened abortion. Dose 10 to 30mg daily.

Dytac. Triamterene, *q.v.*

Dytide. A preparation of triamterene, *q.v.,* and benzthiazide.

E

econazole. An antifungal agent for local application, similar in actions and uses to miconazole, *q.v.*

Ecostatin. Econazole, *q.v.*

ecothiopate. A powerful and long-acting miotic. Strength (0.06 to 0.25%) and frequency of use depend on response. May cause ciliary spasm and headache.

Edecrin. Ethacrynic acid, *q.v.*

edrophonium. A very short-acting drug of the neostigmine type. Used in the diagnosis of myasthenia gravis.

Dose 2 to 10mg by i.v. injection.

Elamol. Tofenacin, *q.v.*

Eldisine. Vindesine, *q.v.*

Eltroxin. Thyroxine, *q.v.*

emepronium. A compound with an atropine-like action on the muscular tone of the urinary bladder. Useful in urinary frequency and tenesmus. Dose 100 to 200mg.

Emeside. Ethosuximide, *q.v.*

emetine. An alkaloid obtained from ipecacuanha, and used in the treatment of acute amoebic dysentery, usually in combination with other amoebicides to obtain maximum effect. Dose 30 to 60mg daily by s.c. or i.m. injection. Also of value in amoebic abscess.

Endoxana. Cyclophosphamide, *q.v.*

Enduron. Methyclothiazide, *q.v.*

enflurane. An inhalation anaesthetic similar to halothane, *q.v.* As with halothane, it may increase the muscle relaxant action of tubocurarine and related drugs. May stimulate CNS, and should not be given in convulsive disorders.

Epanutin. Phenytoin sodium, *q.v.*

ephedrine. A sympathomimetic agent, with a marked relaxant effect on the bronchioles, valuable in the treatment of asthma and bronchial spasm. It also constricts the peripheral vessels, and has been used to counteract the fall in blood pressure that may occur during anaesthesia. Occasionally used in whooping cough, enuresis and as a mydriatic. Care is necessary in hypertension and prostatic enlargement. Dose 15 to 60 mg.

Ephynal. Tocopherol, *q.v.*

Epilim. Sodium valproate, *q.v.*

epinephrine. Adrenaline, *q.v.*

Epodyl. Ethoglucid, *q.v.*

Epontol. Propanidid, *q.v.*

Eppy. A non-irritant solution of adrenaline, *q.v.*, used as eye drops to reduce intra-ocular pressure in glaucoma.

Epsikapron. Aminocaproic acid, *q.v.*

Equanil. Meprobamate, *q.v.*

Eradacin. Acrosoxacin, *q.v.*

ergometrine. The principal alkaloid of ergot, *q.v.* It promotes uterine contraction and is used to control post-partum haemorrhage. Dangerous in the early stages of labour. Dose 0.5 to 1mg orally, or by i.m. injection, smaller doses intravenously.

ergot. A fungus that develops in rye and replaces the normal grain. The active principles include ergometrine, *q.v.*, and ergotamine, *q.v.* Chronic toxic effects characterised by gangrene of the extremities, have followed the use of ergot contaminated rye bread.

ergotamine tartrate. One of the alkaloids of ergot, *q.v.*, but therapeutically it is used solely for the relief of migraine. Early treatment of an impending attack evokes the best response. It should not be used prophylactically owing to the risk of ergotism. Dose 1 to 2mg orally, up to a total of 6mg. It may also be given by oral inhalation.

erythromycin. An orally effective antibiotic, resembling penicillin in its range of activity. Useful in acute streptococcal infections, in pneumonia, and staphylococcal enteritis. It is inactivated by gastric acid, and should be given as coated tablets, or as a suspension of more stable derivatives. In severe infections it may be given by i.v. or i.m. injection. Dose 250mg four times a day.

Esbatal. Bethanidine, *q.v.*

eserine. Physostigmine, *q.v.*

Esidrex. Hydrochlorothiazide, *q.v.* Esidrex-K contains added potassium chloride, to offset the potassium loss in the urine which may occur when treatment is prolonged.

Estracyt. Estramustine, *q.v.*

estramustine. A neoplastic

agent used in prostatic carcinoma. Dose 560mg daily initially, maintenance doses 420 to 840mg daily.

ethacrynic acid. A powerful diuretic with a rapid and intense action. It may be effective when the response to thiazide diuretics is inadequate. May cause, nausea, diarrhoea and deafness. Treatment requires care, as saline loss with hypotension may occur. Initial dose 50mg daily, slowly increased if necessary to a maximum of 400mg daily. Given by i.v. injection in doses of 50mg in acute or refractory oedematous states.

ethambutol. An antitubercular drug, of value in patients hypersensitive or resistant to standard drugs. Dose 15 to 25mg per kg body-weight daily. It may cause visual disturbances requiring withdrawal, and lower doses should be given in renal damage.

ethamivan. A respiratory stimulant similar to nikethamide, *q.v.* Used orally or by injection in respiratory distress in the newborn.

ethamsylate. A systemically effective haemostatic agent used to control bleeding from small blood vessels as in

haematuria, or in surgery. Dose 500mg orally, 250mg by intravenous injection.

ethanolamine oleate. A sclerosing agent used for varicose veins and bleeding oesophageal varices. Dose of injection 2 to 5ml.

ether. A colourless inflammable liquid, once widely used as a general anaesthetic but now largely replaced by halothane, *q.v.* Induction of anaesthesia with ether is unpleasant.

ethinyloestradiol. A synthetic oestrogen more active than stilboestrol, *q.v.*, and with fewer side-effects. Used in menopausal symptoms, amenorrhoea, uterine hypoplasia, functional uterine bleeding, and other conditions where oestrogen therapy is indicated. It is present with a progestogen in many oral contraceptive products. Dose 0.01 to 0.1mg daily. Larger doses are given in prostatic and mammary carcinoma.

ethionamide. An antitubercular drug used as an alternative to isoniazid in the multiple drug treatment of tuberculosis. It is more toxic than isoniazid, and side-effects include nausea and dermatitis. Dose 0.5 to 1g daily.

ethisterone. A synthetic progestogen similar in action to progesterone, but active orally. In amenorrhoea it may be given in association with an oestrogen. Dose 25 to 100mg daily.

ethoglucid. A cytotoxic agent used mainly in bladder papillomatosis by the instillation of a 1% solution.

ethosuximide. An anticonvulsant for the treatment of petit mal epilepsy. May be used alone, or combined with other anticonvulsants, and often of value in patients not responding to other drugs. Dose 250mg daily initially, gradually increased if required to a maximum of 2g daily. Care is necessary in renal or hepatic disease.

ethotoin. An anticonvulsant similar to, but less powerful than phenytoin, *q.v.* Sometimes useful in grand mal not responding to other drugs. Dose 1 to 3g daily.

Ethrane. Enflurane, *q.v.*

ethyl chloride. A volatile anaesthetic used occasionally for induction. It is also a local anaesthetic by virtue of the intense cold produced when sprayed on the skin.

ethyloestrenol. An anabolic steroid with the actions and uses of norethandrolone, *q.v.* Dose 2 to 4mg daily.

etomidate. A drug used mainly for induction of anaesthesia. Dose 0.3mg/kg i.v. Recovery

from a single dose is rapid, but anaesthesia for short procedures can be maintained by additional doses of 0.1 to 0.2mg/kg as required. Intravenous injection requires care, or thrombophlebitis may occur.

Etophylate. Acepifylline, *q.v.*

Eudemine. Diazoxide, *q.v.*

Euglucon. Glibenclamide, *q.v.*

Euhypnos. Temazepam, *q.v.*

Eumavate. Clobetasone, *q.v.*

Eumydrin. Atropine methonitrate, *q.v.*

Eurax. Crotamiton, *q.v.*

eusol. A chlorine antiseptic solution used as lotion, or as compress. The solution should be freshly prepared.

Eutonyl. Pargyline, *q.v.*

F

Fabahistin. Mebhydrolin, *q.v.*

Fanasil. Sulfadoxine, *q.v.*

Fansidar. Pyrimethamine, *q.v.*, 25mg with sulfadoxine, *q.v.*, 500mg. Both these drugs block the formation of folinic acid in the malarial parasite, but the combination is more effective. Of value in patients unable to tolerate chloroquine. Prophylactic dose one tablet weekly. Treatment dose two to three tablets; not to be repeated for at least seven days.

fazadinium. A muscle relaxant

of the tubocurarine (*q.v.*) type, with a rapid action. Used mainly for endotracheal intubation in surgery. Dose 0.75 to 1mg/kg i.v. The action lasts about 40 minutes, but can be reversed by neostigmine.

Fazadon. Fazadinium, *q.v.*

Feldene. Piroxicam, *q.v.*

Femergin. Ergotamine tartrate, *q.v.*

fenbufen. An anti-inflammatory-analgesic agent for the relief of rheumatoid arthritis and similar conditions. Like related drugs it may cause gastric disturbance, rash and dizziness. Dose 600 to 900mg daily.

fenclofenac. An anti-inflammatory drug with an aspirin-like action, but with reduced gastro-intestinal irritant properties. Useful in a wide range of rheumatoid conditions. Dose up to 1200mg daily after food.

fenfluramine. An appetite depressant without the stimulant effects of related drugs. May cause diarrhoea with some patients. Dose 40 to 120mg daily.

fenoprofen. A non-steroidal anti-inflammatory and anti-rheumatic agent. Useful as an alternative drug in rheumatoid arthritis and related conditions. It may cause dizziness, nausea and

intestinal disturbance. Dose 300 to 600mg three or four times a day.

Fenopron. Fenoprofen, *q.v.*

fenoterol. A sympathomimetic agent similar in action to salbutamol, *q.v.* Given by oral inhalation in doses of 0.25mg, up to a maximum of two doses four-hourly.

fentanyl. A morphine-like analgesic, used in association with tranquillisers such as droperidol, *q.v.*, to produce a state of 'neurolepto-analgesia'.

Fentazin. Perphenazine, *q.v.*

feprazone. An anti-inflammatory-analgesic agent with the actions, uses and possible side-effects of phenylbutazone, *q.v.* May be less likely to cause peptic ulceration, but blood dyscrasias may occur. Dose 200 to 600mg daily.

ferrous fumarate, gluconate, sulphate. These compounds are listed under iron, *q.v.*

Flagyl. Metronidazole, *q.v.*

Flamazine. Silver sulphadiazine, *q.v.*

flavoxate. An antispasmodic of value in urinary disorders such as cystitis, urethritis and related conditions. Dose 200mg three times a day. Not recommended for children.

Flaxedil. Gallamine, *q.v.*

Flenac. Fenclofenac, *q.v.*

Florinef. Fludrocortisone, *q.v.*

Floxapen. Flucloxacillin, *q.v.*

flucloxacillin. A derivative of cloxacillin, *q.v.*, but is absorbed more readily when given orally. Dose 250mg six-hourly before meals. In severe infections it may be given by i.m. or i.v. injection.

fludrocortisone. A synthetic steroid with a very powerful salt-retaining action. Valuable in adrenal deficiency state such as Addison's disease, usually to supplement cortisone treatment. Initial dose 1 to 2mg, maintenance dose 0.1 to 0.2mg daily.

flufenamic acid. An analgesic and anti-inflammatory drug of value in rheumatoid, arthritic and other painful conditions. May cause gastric disturbance which can be reduced by divided doses taken after food. Dose 400 to 600mg daily. Use with care in renal disease and peptic ulcer. Contra-indicated in pregnancy.

fluocinolone. A corticosteroid more active by topical application than hydrocortisone. Used as cream, ointment or lotion 0.01 to 0.025%; also with neomycin 0.5% in inflamed and infected skin conditions.

fluocinonide. A locally effective anti-inflammatory steroid similar to fluocinolone, *q.v.*

fluocortolone. A locally active steroid, useful in steroid-responsive eczema and dermatoses.

fluorescein. An orange-red dye; solutions have a strong green fluorescence. Used as eye-drops (2%) for detecting corneal lesions, as areas of cornea denuded of epithelium stain green. Sometimes given by injection to facilitate examination of retinal blood vessels.

fluorouracil. A cytotoxic agent used in the palliative treatment of carcinoma of the breast and gastro-intestinal tract. A standard dose is 12mg/kg daily i.v. for three days, and if tolerated, maintenance doses of 15mg/kg i.v. weekly may be used. A daily dose should not exceed 1g. An oral form (capsules of 250mg) has recently become available for use in multiple therapy, or for long-term maintenance. Side-effects include gastro-intestinal disturbance, leucopenia, alopecia and dermatitis. May cause angina in cardiac patients.

Fluothane. Halothane, *q.v.*

fluoxymesterone. An orally active androgen, used in the palliative treatment of breast cancer, and in osteoporosis as an anabolic agent. Dose 1 to 20mg daily.

flupenthixol. A tranquilliser

similar to fluphenazine, and used in the treatment of schizophrenia. Dose 1 to 4mg daily or 20 to 40mg by deep i.m. injection at intervals of two to four weeks.

fluphenazine. A phenothiazine derivative with more powerful tranquillising and anti-emetic properties than chlorpromazine. Dose 1 to 2mg daily in anxiety states, up to 15mg daily in schizophrenia. A long-acting form for i.m. injection (25mg) has an effect lasting two to three weeks.

flurandrenolone. A potent corticosteroid similar to fluocinolone, *q.v.*, for local use as an anti-inflammatory agent in various skin disorders. Cream and ointment contain 0.0125%.

flurazepam. A non-barbiturate hypnotic similar to nitrazepam, *q.v.* It is of low toxicity, and the risk of 'hangover' effects is slight. Dose 15 to 30mg.

flurbiprofen. An anti-inflammatory agent similar to ibuprofen, *q.v.* Useful in rheumatoid and arthritic conditions. Care is necessary in peptic ulceration, and in aspirin-sensitive asthmatic patients. Dose 150 to 300mg daily.

fluspirilene. A long-acting major tranquilliser, used by i.m. injection in schizophrenia. Dose 2mg weekly initially, average maintenance doses 2 to 8mg weekly. Care is necessary in epilepsy, as it may precipitate seizures.

folic acid. A constituent of the vitamin B group. It is essential for cell division and the growth and development of normal red blood cells. The main use is in the treatment of nutritional macrocytic anaemias, pellagra and tropical sprue. Sometimes given with anti-epileptic drugs, as long-term therapy may cause a folic acid deficiency. Small doses are present in many iron preparations to prevent the megaloblastic anaemia that may occur in later stages of pregnancy. It must not be used in pernicious anaemia, as it cannot prevent the degeneration of the central nervous system associated with that disease. Dose 5 to 20mg; 0.2 to 0.5mg for prophylaxis during pregnancy.

formaldehyde. A powerful but toxic germicide used mainly as 'formalin' in the disinfection of rooms, and as 'formol-saline' (5% in normal saline) for the preservation of pathological specimens. Warts have been treated with a 3% solution.

formalin. A 40% solution of formaldehyde, *q.v.*

Fortral. Pentazocine, *q.v.*

fosfestrol. A water-soluble form of stilboestrol, *q.v.*, used mainly in the treatment of carcinoma of the prostate. Given orally in doses of 100mg or more thrice daily, or by i.v. injection in doses of 500mg or more.

framycetin. An antibiotic resembling neomycin, *q.v.*, in general properties. Used as cream, ointment and lotion. Given by subconjunctival injection in eye infections, and orally for gastro-intestinal infections. Dose 1 to 1.5g.

Framygen. Framycetin, *q.v.*

French chalk. Talc, *q.v.*

friar's balsam. Contains benzoin, storax, aloes, balsam of tolu. Official name Compound Tincture of Benzoin. Used internally and by inhalation in bronchitis, etc., dose 2 to 4ml.

Frisium. Clobazam, *q.v.*

Froben. Flurbiprofen, *q.v.*

frusemide. A diuretic with a powerful and intense action of short duration. Often effective in conditions no longer responding to thiazide diuretics. Dose 40 to 80mg as a single dose, repeated three times a week, or 20mg i.v. injection. Much larger doses may be necessary in renal failure or acute hypertensive crisis. Side-effects include nausea, diarrhoea and cramp. Supplementary potassium is usually necessary as with other powerful diuretics.

Fucidin. Sodium fusidate, *q.v.*

Fulcin. Griseofulvin, *q.v.*

Fungilin. Amphotericin, *q.v.*

Furacin. Nitrofurazone, *q.v.*

Furadantin. Nitrofurantoin, *q.v.*

G

gallamine. A synthetic muscle relaxant with an action similar to that of tubocurarine, *q.v.*, but the effect is less prolonged. Is used extensively in surgery as it is well tolerated, but pre-medication with atropine is necessary to avoid excessive salivation. The action of the drug can be terminated by neostigmine. Average initial dose 80 to 120mg, with small subsequent doses according to need and response. Tachycardia is a side-effect, and may persist longer than the relaxant action.

gammexane. An insecticide similar to DDT, but much more powerful and rapid, and less toxic.

Gantrisin. Sulphafurazole, *q.v.*

Gee's linctus. A soothing cough linctus containing camphorated tincture of opium, oxymel of squill and syrup of tolu. Dose 2 to 4ml.

gentamicin. An antibiotic effective against a wide range of organisms, including *Proteus* and *Pseudomonas*. Of value in septicaemia due to Gram-negative organisms, and may be given with carbenicillin to increase the response. The drug is both nephrotoxic and ototototoxic, and its use requires care. It is not absorbed orally, and for systemic infections is given by i.m. injection in doses of 40 to 80mg. Applied as cream, ointment or drops for local infections.

gentian violet. Crystal violet, *q.v.*

Genticin. Gentamicin, *q.v.*

gestronol. A synthetic progestogen used in the treatment of endometrial carcinoma and benign prostatic hypertrophy. Dose 200 to 400mg by i.m. injection once a week.

glibenclamide. An orally active hypoglycaemic agent, basically similar to chlorpropamide, *q.v.* Effective in doses varying from 2.5 to 20mg daily.

Glibenese. Glipizide, *q.v.*

glibornuride. An orally active hypoglycaemic agent used in late onset diabetes. It is more potent than many related drugs, and is given in doses of 25 to 50mg daily at breakfast.

glipizide. A sulphonylurea, used like tolbutamide, *q.v.*, in diabetes, but effective in much lower doses. Initial dose 5mg, maintenance doses 2.5 to 30mg daily.

gliquidone. An oral hypoglycaemic agent basically similar to chlorpropamide, *q.v.* Effective in maturity-onset diabetes in doses of 40 to 60mg daily, but doses up to 180mg daily have been used.

glucagon. A hormone of the pancreas which raises the blood sugar level by mobilising liver glycogen. Used in insulin hypoglycaemia in doses of 0.5 to 1mg by injection. Large doses by intravenous infusion are sometimes effective in congestive heart failure and cardiac arrhythmia not responding to other drugs.

Glucophage. Metformin, *q.v.*

glucose. Dextrose, *q.v.*

Glurenorm. Gliquidone, *q.v.*

glutaraldehyde. A disinfectant of the formaldehyde (*q.v.*) type, but with a more rapid and powerful action. Effective against a wide range of organisms, including viruses. Used mainly for instrument sterilisation as a 2% solution. Usually activated before use by the addition of a corrosion inhibitor. Such activated solutions are stable for about two weeks.

glutethimide. Hypnotic of medium intensity and duration of action. A useful alternative to the barbiturates. Dose 250 to 500mg at night.

Glutril. Glibornuride, *q.v.*

glycerin, glycerol. A clear syrupy liquid used as a sweetening agent in mixtures and linctuses. It promotes drainage when applied to inflamed areas, and is used as a paste with magnesium sulphate for boils. It is frequently used in the form of suppositories for constipation.

glyceryl trinitrate. A vasodilator used mainly in angina pectoris as tablets 0.5mg, which should be dissolved under the tongue for rapid absorption and prompt effect. A long-acting oral form is available as Sustac. Also given by intravenous infusion to control hypertension and ischaemia during cardiovascular surgery. Dose 10 to 200 micrograms per minute in dextrose-saline. Tolerance may occur with prolonged use, and the drug should be used with care in coronary thrombosis.

glymidine. An oral hypoglycaemic agent, chemically unrelated to tolbutamide, but with a similar action in mild, late-onset diabetes. Initial dose 3g, maintenance dose 0.5 to 1.5g. It may be used with other hypoglycaemic agents.

Gondafon. Glymidine, *q.v.*

gramicidin. A mixture of antibiotics effective against many Gram-positive organisms, but it is too toxic for systemic use. Used topically in infected skin conditions, usually in association with neomycin and hydrocortisone.

griseofulvin. An orally active antifungal antibiotic. It is deposited selectively in the skin, hair and nails, and prevents further fungal invasion. Widely used in ringworm and tinea infections, but prolonged treatment is necessary. May cause headache, allergic reactions and gastric disturbance. Dose 0.5 to 1g daily.

Grisovin. Griseofulvin, *q.v.*

guanethidine. A valuable antihypertensive drug with a powerful and prolonged action. It brings about a smooth reduction in blood-pressure by blocking transmission in adrenergic nerves, and preventing the release of noradrenaline, *q.v.* It is widely employed in the treatment of all types of hypertension, often with a thiazide diuretic. Dose 10mg daily, increased by 10mg at weekly intervals according to response, with average doses of 50 to 75mg daily, although sometimes much larger doses are required. Diarrhoea, weakness and bradycardia are common side-effects. Guanethidine is occasionally used as eyedrops in glaucoma and thyrotoxicosis.

guanoclor. An antihypertensive drug with an action similar to that of guanethidine, *q.v.* Dose 10 to 20mg daily as necessary up to 40mg daily. Occasionally much larger doses may be required. Care is necessary in hepatic dysfunction.

guanoxan. An antihypertensive drug similar in action to guanethidine, *q.v.* Useful in hypertension not responding to other drugs, but liver damage has been reported. Dose 10 to 50mg daily.

H

Haelan. Flurandrenolone, *q.v.*

Halcion. Triazolam, *q.v.*

halibut-liver oil. A rich source of vitamins A and D. Dose 0.2 to 0.5ml.

haloperidol. A tranquilliser chemically unrelated to chlorpromazine, but having a basically similar but longer action. Valuable in mania and schizophrenic excitement. Dose 3 to 9mg or more daily.

halothane. A widely used inhalation anaesthetic, more powerful and less toxic than ether or chloroform, with the advantage of not being inflammable. It suppresses mucous and bronchial secretions, and reduces capillary bleeding. Suxamethonium is preferred if increased muscle relaxation is required. Hepatic damage has followed the use of halothane; the association is not clear, but care is necessary in patients with liver dysfunction. May cause bradycardia and cardiac irregularity.

Harmonyl. Deserpidine, *q.v.*

Hartmann's solution. An electrolyte replacement solution containing sodium lactate, sodium chloride, potassium chloride, and calcium chloride; given orally or intravenously in acidosis and gastroenteritis.

Heminevrin. Chlormethiazole, *q.v.*

heparin. The natural anticoagulant obtained from lung and liver tissue. It is widely used in the treatment of postoperative thrombosis and thromboembolic diseases. It is given by i.v. injection and the action is prompt but brief, so four-hourly injections are necessary to maintain the effect. Toxic reactions are few and slight.

Dose 5000 to 15 000 units. Intramuscular injections are painful and less reliable. Overdosage can be controlled by i.v. injection of protamine sulphate, *q.v.* Treatment with heparin may be combined with that of oral anticoagulants such as phenindione, *q.v.*, or warfarin, *q.v.*, to provide immediate action before the slow-acting oral drugs begin to take effect. Given for prophylaxis against thrombosis in a dose of 5000 units s.c., pre-operatively, and similar doses post-operation eight-hourly for seven days.

heroin. Diamorphine, *q.v.*

Herpid. Idoxuridine, *q.v.*

hexachlorophane. An antiseptic used for skin sterilisation, and present in some medicated soaps.

hexamine. A formaldehyde derivative of low toxicity, occasionally used as a urinary antiseptic. Usually given as Hiprex, *q.v.*, or Mandelamine, *q.v.*

Hexopal. Inositol nicotinate, *q.v.*

Hibitane. Chlorhexidine, *q.v.*

Hiprex. A compound of hexamine, *q.v.*, and hippuric acid that provides the acidification of the urine necessary for hexamine to have an antibacterial action. Of value in chronic urinary infections,

and for prophylaxis before and after urological surgery.

histamine. A compound present in a bound form in all mammalian tissues; its release is probably the ultimate cause of many allergic conditions. It has been used in circulatory disorders. Dose 0.5 to 1mg by s.c. or i.m. injection.

Histryl. Diphenylpyraline, *q.v.*

homatropine. An atropine derivative with a similar but more rapid mydriatic action (15 to 30 minutes), but a shorter duration of effect. Solution (2%) is often used with cocaine, which increases the effect.

Honvan. Fosfesterol, *q.v.*

Hyalase. Hyaluronidase, *q.v.*

hyaluronidase. A 'spreading' factor derived from testes. When intravenous drip infusion of an electrolyte solution is impracticable, the injection of 1mg of hyaluronidase will promote the absorption of 500 to 1000ml of electrolyte solution by *subcutaneous* drip infusion.

hydralazine. A synthetic drug with useful antihypertensive properties mainly by direct peripheral vasodilation. It is given in essential and malignant hypertension, usually in association with a thiazide diuretic. Dose 12.5mg initially, four times a day, slowly increased to 200mg daily as required. Also given by intravenous drip in doses of 20 to 40mg in hypertensive emergencies such as pre-eclampsia.

hydrargaphen. An organic mercurial compound with antibacterial and antifungal properties. Used for skin preparation, and as pessaries for vaginitis.

Hydrea. Hydroxyurea, *q.v.*

Hydrenox. Hydroflumethiazide, *q.v.*

hydrochlorothiazide. A widely used thiazide diuretic. It brings about a marked increase in the excretion of salts and water, and is of considerable value in congestive heart failure, and other oedematous conditions. The drug increases the excretion of potassium as well as sodium, and if treatment is prolonged, some potassium replacement therapy will be necessary, such as potassium chloride, *q.v.*, or as effervescent potassium tablets. Hydrochlorothiazide is also useful in hypertension as it potentiates the action of other drugs. Dose 25 to 50mg.

hydrocortisone. A derivative of cortisone, *q.v.*, with marked anti-inflammatory effects, particularly when applied locally. Widely employed in inflammatory skin, eye and ear conditions, sometimes in association with antibiotics such as neomycin, to reduce secondary bacterial invasion. Ointments should be applied thinly in strengths from 0.5 to 1%. Frequently given by intra-articular injection in bursitis and associated conditions. Of great value in status asthmaticus, allergic emergencies and shock-like states when given i.v. in doses of 100mg. Also given orally in deficiency states in doses varying from 10 to 40mg or more.

hydroflumethiazide. A diuretic similar in action and uses to hydrochlorothiazide, *q.v.* Dose 25 to 100mg.

hydrogen peroxide solution. Contains 5 to 7% H_2O_2, giving about 20 volumes of oxygen. A deodorising antiseptic used mainly for cleaning wounds. Also used as a mouthwash (diluted 1 to 7) and ear drops (1 in 4 in water or 50% alcohol).

HydroSaluric. Hydrochlorothiazide, *q.v.*

hydroxocobalamin. A drug closely related to cyanocobalamin, *q.v.*, but is excreted much more slowly. Adequate blood levels in pernicious and megaloblastic anaemia can be maintained by a monthly injection of 250 micrograms.

hydroxyprogesterone. A progesterone derivative given by i.m. injection of an oily solution. Mainly used in the first half of pregnancy to reduce the risk of abortion. Dose 250 to 500mg weekly.

hydroxyurea. A cytotoxic agent sometimes used instead of busulphan in myeloid leukaemia. Also used in some superficial cancers. Dose 20 to 30mg/kg as a single dose daily, or 80mg/kg as a single dose every third day.

hydroxyzine. A minor tranquilliser and anti-emetic. Useful in anxiety and agitation, and as a sedative in dermatoses complicated by emotional tension. Not recommended in pregnancy, or where sedation is undesirable. Dose 75 to 300mg daily.

Hygroton. Chlorthalidone, *q.v.*

hyoscine. Also known as scopolamine. An alkaloid obtained from plants of the belladonna group. It is a powerful hypnotic and is widely used together with papaveretum for pre-medication before operation. Also has anti-emetic properties, and is useful in travel sickness. Dose 0.3 to 0.6mg.

hyoscine butylbromide. A derivative of hyoscine that resembles atropine in its antispasmodic action, but differs in lacking any action on the central nervous system. Useful in spasm and hypermotility of the gastro-intestinal tract. Dose 10 to 20mg.

Hypnomidate. Etomidate, *q.v.*

Hypovase. Prazosin, *q.v.*

hypromellose. A water-soluble cellulose derivative used in some ophthalmic products. It forms the basis of 'artificial tears', and extends the action of medicated eye drops.

I

ibuprofen. An anti-inflammatory and analgesic agent widely used in the treatment of rheumatoid arthritis and similar conditions. Is generally well tolerated if taken after meals, but care is necessary in peptic ulcer, liver dysfunction and asthma. Dose 1200mg daily initially, adjusted to maintenance doses of 600mg or more.

ichthammol. A thick, dark brown liquid with a characteristic odour, derived from certain bituminous oils. It is a mild antiseptic and is used in ointments, and as solution (10%) in glycerin for ulcers and inflamed areas.

idoxuridine. An antiviral agent

used locally in dendritic ulcers of the eye as drops of 0.1% solution or 0.5% ointment. Also applied as a 5% solution in dimethyl sulphoxide in herpes zoster skin infections. Has also been used intravenously for systemic viral infections.

ifosfamide. A derivative of cyclophosphamide, *q.v.*, but much more toxic. Usually given in association with other cytotoxic drugs. Total dose 8 to 10g/square metre, divided into single daily doses over 3 to 10 days, and given by intravenous infusion. Adequate diuresis is essential, as the drug may cause very severe renal toxicity.

Ilotycin. Erythromycin, *q.v.*

Imferon. An iron-dextran preparation for i.m. injection. Used in iron-deficiency anaemias when oral iron preparations are not tolerated. Dose 5ml daily, or on alternate days, according to degree of haemoglobin deficiency. The total amount so required is occasionally given as a single dose by slow intravenous drip infusion, but reactions have followed such total dose infusions.

imipramine. A tricyclic psychotherapeutic drug with powerful and specific antidepressant properties. Response to the drug may be slow, and long treatment is often necessary. Dose 25mg three times a day, gradually increased to 50mg as required. Some side-effects are anticholinergic in character, but the drug is contraindicated in liver damage or ischaemic heart disease. Imipramine should not be given in association with or soon after monoamine oxidase inhibitors, as the effects of both drugs may be increased.

Imodium. Loperamide, *q.v.*

Imperacin. Oxytetracycline, *q.v.*

Imuran. Azathioprine, *q.v.*

indapamide. A drug with a slow but progressive antihypertensive action. Given in doses of 2.5mg daily, continued for some months, until a maximum response has been obtained. Larger doses do not evoke an increased hypotensive response, but may have a diuretic action. The response may be increased by combined treatment with beta-blocking agents and related drugs if required, but the use of saluretic diuretics is not recommended.

Inderal. Propranolol, *q.v.*

indigo carmine. A blue dye used as a 0.4% solution by injection as a renal function test. Normally the urine is coloured blue in 10 minutes or so.

Indocid. Indomethacin, *q.v.*

indomethacin. An anti-inflammatory and analgesic drug of value in many arthritic and rheumatoid conditions, and in acute gout. Administration as suppository gives a prolonged action, and is useful at night to reduce morning stiffness. Side-effects include headache, nausea and dyspepsia, and blood disorders may occur. Care is necessary in renal and hepatic disease. Dose 50 to 150mg daily; 100mg as suppository.

indoramin. An alpha-adrenoceptor blocking agent used in hypertension. Can be added to existing thiazide treatment, or used with a beta blocking agent. Drowsiness is an occasional side-effect. Dose 25mg twice a day, adjusted at weekly intervals. Maximum daily dose 200mg.

inositol nicotinate. A peripheral vasodilator similar to tolazoline, *q.v.* Dose 400mg to 1g.

insulin. The antidiabetic principle of the pancreas, regulating the metabolism of carbohydrates and fats. It is widely used by s.c. injection in the treatment of diabetes mellitus. Many modified insulin products, such as the 'Lente' and MC (monocomponent) insulins are now available, designed to extend the action of the drug, reduce the frequency of injections, and so simulate the effects of the natural hormone more closely. Dosage is based entirely on the patient's requirements. In diabetic emergency, soluble insulin remains the preparation of choice.

Intal. Sodium cromoglycate, *q.v.*

Integrin. Oxypertine, *q.v.*

Intralipid. An emulsion of soya oil, specially prepared for slow intravenous injection when a high calorie intake is required, as in severe malnutrition.

Intraval Sodium. Thiopentone sodium, *q.v.*

Intropin. Dopamine, *q.v.*

iodine. Powerful antiseptic used as iodine solution, or as povidone-iodine, *q.v.*, for skin preparation. Allergic reactions to iodine skin applications are not unknown. Given orally as Lugol's solution, *q.v.*, in pre-operative treatment of thyrotoxicosis. Dose: as Aqueous Iodine Solution (Lugol's Solution) 0.1 to 1ml; as Weak Iodine Solution (tincture of iodine) 0.6 to 2ml.

iodised oil. Poppy-seed oil containing 40% iodine in combination. Used as contrast agent in x-ray examination of bronchial tract, uterus, fistulae, etc. The oil decomposes and darkens slowly on storage, and only colourless or pale yellow material should be used.

iodoform. Yellow powder with strong odour. Mild antiseptic used occasionally as BIPP, *q.v.*

iopanoic acid. A radio-opaque substance used as a contrast agent in cholecystography. It is largely excreted in the bile when given orally. Dose 2 to 6g.

ipecacuanha. The dried root from which emetine, *q.v.*, is obtained. It has expectorant and emetic properties, and is used mainly as the tincture. Dose 0.25 to 1ml; emetic dose, 5 to 20ml.

ipratropium. An anticholinergic agent with bronchodilator properties. Given by oral inhalation in bronchospasm. Dose 18 to 36 micrograms three or four times a day.

iprindole. A tricyclic antidepressant with uses and side-effects similar to those of imipramine, *q.v.* Dose 45 to 90mg daily.

iproniazid. A monoamine oxidase inhibitor with the antidepressant action, uses and side-effects of phenelzine, *q.v.* Dose 50 to 100mg daily.

iron gluconate. Ferrous gluconate. One of the most widely used preparations for iron-deficiency anaemias. It is less irritating than ferrous sulphate and is a useful alternative when the sulphate is not tolerated. Prophylactic dose 600mg daily; therapeutic dose 2.4 to 4.8g daily.

iron sulphate. Ferrous sulphate. Used extensively in iron-deficiency anaemias as it is effective in small doses, and fairly well tolerated but may cause gastric disturbance in some patients. Usually given as tablets, each containing 200mg. These tablets are potentially dangerous for small children as death has occurred after accidental administration.

Ismelin. Guanethidine, *q.v.*

isocarboxazid. A monoamine oxidase inhibitor, *q.v.*, used in the treatment of depression. Dose 30mg initially daily, reduced later to 10 to 20mg according to need.

isoetharine. A bronchodilator similar to isoprenaline, *q.v.*, but with a longer action. Dose 10 to 30mg daily.

Isogel. Red granules of mucilage from various seeds, for use as a bulk-increasing laxative. Dose 2 to 4g or more.

isoniazid. A pyridine derivative with a specific action against *Mycobacterium tuberculosis.* Widely used in the treatment of tuberculosis, but as bacterial resistance soon develops, combined treatment with other antitubercular drugs is essential. Side-effects include nausea and peripheral neuritis. Dose 300 to 600mg daily.

isoprenaline. A compound closely related to adrenaline, *q.v.*, but with increased bronchodilator and reduced vaso-constrictor potency. Widely used in asthma, bronchospasm, etc., by oral inhalation from special aerosol inhalers, or as sublingual tablets (20mg). Side-effects include tachycardia and nausea.

isopropyl alcohol. Colourless inflammable liquid. Used for pre-operative skin preparation, and also as solvent for iodine-containing skin products in preference to industrial alcohol.

Isordil. Isosorbide dinitrate, *q.v.*

isosorbide dinitrate. A vasodilator with a more prolonged action than glyceryl trinitrate, *q.v.* Used prophylactically in angina in doses of 5 to 20mg two or three times a day. Used sublingually in acute attacks of angina.

isoxuprine. A peripheral vasodilator used in some circulatory disorders in doses of 30 to 80mg daily. It also inhibits uterine contractions, and has been given by intravenous infusion in doses of 100mg to control premature labour. Side-effects include transient flushing, tachycardia and hypotension.

J

Jectofer. A soluble complex of iron, sorbitol, citric acid and dextrin. Used by i.m. injection in iron-deficiency anaemias in doses of 2ml daily, the total dose being based on the degree of haemoglobin deficiency.

K

kanamycin. An antibiotic related to neomycin, *q.v.*, but less toxic and so suitable for systemic use. It is given by intramuscular injection in severe infections due to Gram-negative and Gram-positive organisms particularly those resistant to other antibiotics. Dose 1 to 2g daily in divided doses, carefully adjusted to avoid neurotoxic reactions and possible deafness. Some reversible kidney damage is relatively common. Occasionally given orally like neomycin, q.v., in intestinal infections.

Kannasyn. Kanamycin, q.v.

kaolin. Aluminium silicate. Used as an adsorbent in diarrhoea, colitis, food poisoning, etc. often as Kaolin and Morphine Mixture, and as a dusting powder. Dose 15 to 50g.

Kefadol. Cefamandole, q.v.

Keflex. Cephalexin, q.v.

Keflin. Cephalothin, q.v.

Kefzol. Cephazolin, q.v.

Kelfizine. Sulfametopyrazine, q.v.

Kelocyanor. A specific antidote for cyanide poisoning. Contains dicobalt edetate, and when given intravenously, binds any cyanide in the blood. Dose 300mg by slow i.v. injection. Adverse reactions may occur if given in the absence of cyanide, as in misdiagnosis.

Kemadrin. Procyclidine, q.v.

Kenalog. Triamcinolone, q.v.

Kerecid. Idoxuridine, q.v.

Ketalar. Ketamine, q.v.

ketamine. A short-acting intravenous anaesthetic with analgesic properties. It is given in doses of 2mg per kg body-weight, and produces anaesthesia in about 30 seconds, which lasts 5 to 10 minutes. The analgesic action of ketamine is useful in certain neurodiagnostic procedures, and in the treatment of severe burns. Care should be taken not to disturb the patient during the post-anaesthetic period, as vivid dreams or hallucinations may occur during the recovery phase.

Kethamed. Pemoline, q.v.

ketoconazole. A broad spectrum, orally active antimycotic agent. Of value in deep mycoses, and superficial mycoses that have not responded to local treatment. Dose 200 to 400mg daily with food, continued for a week after clearance of symptoms.

ketoprofen. An anti-inflammatory and analgesic agent used in rheumatoid arthritis, gout, spondylitis and related conditions. Generally well tolerated, but should be given with food. Care is necessary in peptic ulcer and hepatic disease. May increase the action of anticoagulants and other drugs bound to plasma protein. Like aspirin, it is an inhibitor of prostaglandin synthesis. Dose 100 to 200 mg daily.

ketotifen. An inhibitor of histamine release, with an action recalling that of sodium cromoglycate, q.v. It has the great advantage of being active orally, and is indicated in the prophylaxis of asthma. Dose 1 to 2mg twice daily with food, continued for some weeks to obtain maximum response. Of no value in attacks of asthma.

Konakion. Phytomenadione, *q.v.*

L

labetalol. A beta-blocking agent, *q.v.*, with some alpha-blocking activity. Useful in all grades of hypertension. Should be used with care in asthmatics, and AV block is a contra-indication. Initial dose 100mg three times a day, slowly increasing as required to a maximum of 2 to 4g daily.

lactic acid. The acid present in sour milk. Used mainly as Compound Sodium Lactate Injection in acidosis and electrolyte disturbances. The injection solution is sometimes given orally in infantile gastro-enteritis. Calcium lactate sometimes used in calcium replacement therapy.

lactoflavin. Riboflavine, *q.v.*

lactulose. A sugar that is not absorbed by the gastrointestinal tract. Used in the treatment of chronic constipation and hepatic encephalopathy. Dose 5 to 20g daily.

laevulose (fructose). An easily digested sugar, particularly for diabetes as it can be converted to glycogen in the absence of insulin. Sometimes given intravenously as an alternative to dextrose.

Lamprene. Clofazimine, *q.v.*

lanatoside C. A cardiac glycoside from *Digitalis lanata*. It is excreted more rapidly than some digitalis products and so has a wider margin of safety. Dose 1 to 1.5mg orally, for rapid digitalisation, followed by maintenance doses of 0.25 to 0.75mg daily.

Lanitop. Medigoxin, *q.v.*

lanolin. Wool fat.

Lanoxin. Digoxin, *q.v.*

Lanvis. Thioguanine, *q.v.*

Largactil. Chlorpromazine, *q.v.*

Larodopa. Levodopa, *q.v.*

Lasix. Frusemide, *q.v.*

Lassar's paste. A stiff ointment containing zinc oxide, starch and white soft paraffin with 2% salicylic acid. Used as protective in eczema.

laudanum. Tincture of opium; contains morphine 1%. Dose 0.3 to 2ml.

Laxoberal. Sodium picosulphate, *q.v.*

Ledercort. Triamcinolone, *q.v.*

Lederfen. Fenbufen, *q.v.*

Lederkyn. Sulphamethoxypyridazine, *q.v.*

Ledermycin. Demeclocycline, *q.v.*

Lenium. Selenium sulphide, *q.v.*

Lentizol. Amitriptyline, *q.v.*

Leukeran. Chlorambucil, *q.v.*

levallorphan. A morphine antagonist which in small doses is claimed to inhibit the respiratory depression induced by morphine and related drugs.

levodopa. An amino-acid that is converted to dopamine in the body. It is used in the treatment of Parkinson's disease, which is associated with a reduction in brain dopamine levels due to degeneration in the corpus striatum. Side-effects include nausea, dizziness and psychiatric disturbance. Dose 0.5g daily initially, slowly increasing according to response to 6 to 9g daily.

levonorgestrel. Norgestrel, *q.v.*

Levophed. Solution of noradrenaline, *q.v.*, for treatment of shock. Given by slow intravenous injection after 1:250 dilution with saline.

levorphanol. Powerful analgesic similar to morphine, effective both orally and by injection. Tablets of 1.5mg, ampoules of 2mg, for i.m. or s.c. injection.

Librium. Chlordiazepoxide, *q.v.*

lidoflazine. A coronary vaso-dilator used in angina. Dose 120mg daily, increasing at weekly intervals to 120mg three times a day.

lignocaine. A local anaesthetic similar to procaine, but with a more intense and extended effect. Used for infiltration anaesthesia as 0.5 to 2% solution, usually with adrenaline. Widely used in dentistry. A 2 to 4% solution is used for local application before bronchoscopy. It reduces cardiac irritability, and is given in doses of 50 to 100mg by slow intravenous injection, to control ventricular arrhythmias following cardiac infarction.

Limclair. Sodium edetate, *q.v.*

Lincocin. Lincomycin, *q.v.*

lincomycin. An orally active antibiotic with a range of activity similar to that of erythromycin. Well absorbed and widely distributed in tissues, bone and pleural fluids, and excreted in urine. Dose 500mg four times a day before meals; in severe conditions 600mg or more twice daily by i.m. or i.v. injection.

Lioresal. Baclofen, *q.v.*

liothyronine. A hormone of the thyroid gland with a rapid action, and probably the substance into which thyroxine, *q.v.*, is converted. Useful in patients not responding to thyroxine. Dose 5 to 100 micrograms daily.

Lipiodol. Iodised oil, *q.v.*

lithium carbonate. Used in the prophylaxis of manic-depressive disease. The mode of action is not known but careful control of the plasma lithium level is necessary to avoid toxic side-effects. Dose 0.25 to 1.5g daily.

Lomodex. Dextran, *q.v.*

Lomotil. A preparation of diphenoxylate, *q.v.*, used in doses of two tablets six-hourly for the control of diarrhoea.

lomustine. An orally active cytotoxic drug used in Hodgkin's disease and solid tumours. Dose 130mg per square metre of body surface every six weeks. Toxic effects include anorexia, nausea, leucopenia and liver damage.

Loniten. Minoxidil, *q.v.*

loperamide. A synthetic inhibitor of peristalsis, of value in the treatment of acute diarrhoea. Dose 4mg initially, followed by three or four doses of 2mg to a maximum daily dose of 16mg.

Lopresor. Metoprolol, *q.v.*

lorazepam. An antidepressant useful in anxiety and tension states not responding to other drugs. Dose 1 to 10mg daily.

Lorfan. Levallorphan, *q.v.*

Lucidril. Meclofenoxate, *q.v.*

Ludiomil. Maprotiline, *q.v.*

Lugol's solution. An aqueous solution of iodine 5%, potassium iodide 10%. Used in the pre-operative treatment of thyrotoxicosis. Dose 0.3 to 1ml.

Luminal. Phenobarbitone, *q.v.*

lymecycline. A soluble complex of tetracycline, *q.v.*, and lysine. It has the action and uses of tetracycline, but is absorbed more readily, giving higher blood levels of the antibiotic.

lynoestrenol. A progestogen similar to norethisterone, *q.v.* A constituent of some oral contraceptive products.

Lynoral. Ethinyloestradiol, *q.v.*

lysol. A solution of cresol, *q.v.*, 50% in a liquid soap. It is a powerful but caustic disinfectant, but care must be taken that it does not come in contact with the skin. Related but less caustic preparations are represented by Sudol and Clearsol.

M

Macrodantin. Nitrofurantoin, *q.v.*

Macrodex. Dextran, *q.v.*

Madopar. A preparation of levodopa, *q.v.*, and benserazide, *q.v.*, for parkinsonism.

Madribon. Sulphadimethoxine, *q.v.*

magnesium carbonate. A white, insoluble powder with antacid and laxative properties. Dose 0.6 to 4g.

magnesium hydroxide. A mild antacid laxative, usually given in aqueous suspension as Cream of Magnesia, although tablet forms are also available. It is often preferred to magnesium carbonate, as no release of carbon dioxide and consequent gastric distension follows its use. Cream of Magnesia is a useful antidote in mineral acid poisoning.

magnesium sulphate (Epsom salts). A powerful saline aperient, producing loose stools by preventing the reabsorption of water. Used externally for the treatment of boils and carbuncles as a paste with glycerin.

magnesium trisilicate. A white insoluble powder, with mild but prolonged antacid effects. It is widely employed for the treatment of peptic ulcer, often in association with other antacids. Dose 0.3 to 2g.

malathion. An organophosphorus insecticide. Used as a lotion 0.5% for lice and scabies as alternative to dicophane, *q.v.*

Malaprim. Tablets of pyrimethamine 12.5mg and dapsone 100mg, for chloroquine-resistant malaria. Dose one tablet weekly.

Mandelamine. Hexamine mandelate, referred to under hexamine, *q.v.*

mandelic acid. Used as ammonium or hexamine mandelate as a bacteriostat in *E. coli* infections of the urinary tract when more powerful drugs are not tolerated.

Mandl's paint. A solution of iodine in glycerin. Used occasionally in tonsillitis as an antiseptic throat paint.

mannitol. A sugar that is not metabolised, and is used mainly as an osmotic diuretic. It is given by slow intravenous injection in doses of 100g as a 10 or 20% solution to reduce cerebral oedema; useful for increasing urinary elimination in drug overdose. Care is necessary to maintain fluid balance. Also used to determine the glomerular filtration rate.

maprotiline. A *tetra*-cyclic antidepressant, but in many ways it resembles the tricyclic antidepressants such as imipramine, *q.v.* It also has sedative properties. Dose 25 to 150mg daily. If given at night as a single dose, the sedative action may reduce the need for other drugs.

Marcain. Bupivacaine, *q.v.*

Marevan. Warfarin, *q.v.*

Marplan. Isocarboxazid, *q.v.*

Marsilid. Iproniazid, *q.v.*

Marzine. Cyclizine, *q.v.*

Masteril. Drostanolone, *q.v.*

Maxolon. Metoclopramide, *q.v.*

mazindol. An appetite depressant for use in obesity. Care is necessary if used with anti-hypertensive drugs, and antidepressants of the monoamine oxidase inhibitor type. Dose 2mg daily after breakfast.

mebendazole. An anthelmintic effective against most intestinal worms. Given as a single dose of 100mg for threadworm, and 100mg twice daily for two days against other infestations. Generally well tolerated.

mebeverine. An anti-spasmodic with a direct action on colonic smooth muscle. Useful in gastro-intestinal spasm. Dose 100mg four times a day before food.

mebhydrolin. An antihistamine used in hayfever, urticaria and other allergic conditions. Dose 50 to 100mg three times a day.

mecillinam. An antibiotic that is active mainly against *E. coli*, *Proteus*, *Shigella*, *Salmonella* and related organisms. Much less active against Gram-positive organisms; Pseudomonas is highly resistant. Useful in some urinary infections and typhoid fever. Dose 5mg/kg, i.m. or slow i.v. injection six- to eight-hourly. In severe infections, 10 to 15mg/kg six-hourly. Care is necessary in renal dysfunction.

meclofenoxate. A central stimulant, used in mental confusion, depression and melancholia, and in delirium tremens. Has also been used in anoxia and coma. Dose 300mg four times a day.

medazepam. A tranquillising agent similar to chlordiazepoxide, *q.v.* Used in anxiety and tension states, and in alcoholism. Dose 15 to 40mg daily.

medigoxin. A derivative of digoxin, *q.v.*, but effective in lower doses. 300 micrograms is said to be equivalent to 500 micrograms of digoxin.

Medrone. Methylprednisolone, *q.v.*

medroxyprogesterone. Has the actions and uses of progesterone, *q.v.*, but is also active orally. Dose 10 to 30mg daily for some weeks to inhibit abortion; 2.5 to 10mg daily for menstrual disorders; 200 to 400mg daily in some hormone-dependent cancers. Given by i.m. injection in doses of 50mg weekly for endometriosis.

mefenamic acid. An analgesic drug with anti-inflammatory properties, useful in arthritis and rheumatoid conditions. May cause gastro-intestinal disturbance. Dose 250mg four times a day.

Mefoxin. Cefoxitin, *q.v.*

mefruside. A diuretic with a slower and more prolonged action than related drugs such as frusemide, *q.v.* Useful in the long-term treatment of oedema, in hypertension and pre-menstrual tension. Dose 12.5 to 50mg daily, according to need and response. A potassium supplement may be required. Care is necessary in renal and hepatic deficiency.

Megaclor. Clomocycline, *q.v.*

Megimide. Bemegride, *q.v.*

melarsoprol. A trypanocide used in late trypanosomiasis as an alternative to tryparsamide, *q.v.* Suitable for hospital use only.

Melleril. Thioridazine, *q.v.*

melphalan. A cytostatic drug with an action similar to mustine, *q.v.* Used in multiple myeloma, and by isolated perfusion in malignant melanoma. Oral dose 10 to 30mg; by perfusion 70 to 100mg.

menadiol. A water-soluble synthetic vitamin K, *q.v.* Used in prophylaxis of haemorrhagic disorders, dose 5 to 10mg; in obstetrics before delivery, 5 to 10mg, i.m. For treatment, phytomenadione, *q.v.*, is preferred.

menotrophin. Human menopausal gonadotrophin containing follicle-stimulating hormone and luteinising hormone. Used in anovulatory sterility and to stimulate spermatogenesis. Dose depends on hormone assays, and individual need and response.

menthol. Colourless crystals obtained from oil of peppermint. Used as spray or drops for naso-pharyngeal inflammation, and as an inhalation, often with friar's balsam, for the relief of coryza and catarrh.

mepacrine. A synthetic antimalarial. Now replaced by chloroquine, *q.v.*, proguanil, *q.v.*, and other powerful antimalarial drugs.

mepivacaine. A local anaesthetic similar to lignocaine, *q.v.* It has no vasodilator action, and may be used without the addition of adrenaline.

meprobamate. A mild tranquillising drug. Indicated in neurotic and tension states, alcoholism and associated conditions. It may cause allergic skin reactions and bronchospasm in sensitive patients. Dose 400mg three to four times a day.

mepyramine maleate. One of the less potent antihistamines. It is used in allergic conditions such as urticaria, hayfever and drug reactions.

It has antipruritic and local analgesic properties; useful as cream in pruritus and insect bites and stings. Extended local use may cause skin sensitisation.

mequitazine. An antihistamine which causes less sedation than promethazine, *q.v.* Dose 5mg twice a day.

Meralen. Flufenamic acid, *q.v.*

Merbentyl. Dicyclomine, *q.v.*

mercaptopurine. A cytotoxic agent used in the treatment of acute leukaemia and chronic myelogenous leukaemia. The best results are obtained in children. Close haematological control throughout treatment is essential. Dose 2.5mg per kg body-weight daily.

mercurochrome. A red dye with weak antiseptic properties. Used occasionally for skin sterilisation.

Merital. Nomifensine, *q.v.*

Merthiolate. Thiomersal, *q.v.*

Mesontoin. Methoin, *q.v.*

mesterolone. An orally active androgen with the actions and uses of testosterone, *q.v.* Dose 50 to 100mg daily.

Mestinon. Pyridostigmine, *q.v.*

mestranol. An orally active oestrogen, with the actions and uses of oestradiol, *q.v.* Used mainly in association with a progestogen. Present in many oral contraceptive products.

metaraminol. A vasopressor drug with a powerful and prolonged action. Of great value in the hypotension of shock, haemorrhage, myocardial infarction and infection. Is suitable for intramuscular or subcutaneous injection as unlike noradrenaline it does not cause local tissue damage. May also be given by slow intravenous drip infusion after dilution with saline or dextrose solution. Dose 2 to 10mg.

metformin. An orally active hypoglycaemic agent similar in action to phenformin, *q.v.* Dose 1.5g daily, adjusted according to need and response.

methacycline. A tetracycline, *q.v.*, derivative with the general antibacterial action of that group of drugs. Dose 600 to 1200mg daily.

methadone. A synthetic analgesic resembling morphine in its general effects, but its sedative action is less marked. It is also a cough centre depressant and is of value in the treatment of severe and useless cough, but great care is necessary with children, as they can tolerate small doses only. Dose 5 to 10mg orally, or by s.c. or i.m. injection.

methandienone. A non-virilising androgen, used in osteoporosis and protein deficiency states. Care is necessary in liver dysfunction and in prostatic disturbances. Dose 5 to 10mg.

methicillin. A penicillin derivative active against penicillinase-producing staphylococci, but less active against other organisms. Its use has declined as other and orally active penicillins such as flucloxacillin (*q.v.*) have become available. Dose 1g i.m. four- to six-hourly. Used in ophthalmic surgery in doses of 500mg by subconjunctival injection.

methionine. A sulphur-containing amino-acid essential for nutrition. It has been used in toxic hepatitis and to increase the effects of some urinary antiseptics by increasing the acidity of the urine. Dose 3 to 10g daily. Also used in paracetamol poisoning in doses of 2.5g four-hourly up to a total of 10g, orally or i.v., as an alternative to acetylcysteine, *q.v.*

methixene. A drug with mild anticholinergic and antihistaminic properties. Used in the treatment of parkinsonism, but relieves the tremor more than the rigidity. It may be given with other drugs to evoke a full response. Dose 15 to 60mg daily.

methocarbamol. A skeletal muscle relaxant used in fibrositis and rheumatic states. Dose 4g daily.

methohexitone. An intravenous anaesthetic similar to thiopentone, *q.v.*, but with a very short action and quick recovery rate. Used for induction anaesthesia or minor operations. Dose 50 to 120mg.

methoin. An anticonvulsant similar to phenytoin, used mainly in the treatment of grand mal. Side-effects more frequent than with phenytoin, and blood changes may also occur. Care is necessary in allergic patients. Dose 100 to 600mg daily.

methoserpidine. A derivative of reserpine, *q.v.*, used in the treatment of hypertension. Dose 30mg or more daily.

methotrexate. A folic acid antagonist and cytotoxic agent used in acute lymphatic leukaemia. Given in daily oral doses of 3mg per square metre body surface, or doses of 15mg per square metre orally or by injection once a week. Larger doses of 20 to 100mg per square metre by intravenous infusion in bronchial and other carcinomas. Close control of blood count and liver function essential. Side-effects common, and include nausea, mouth ulceration, kidney and liver damage. It has also been used in resistant psoriasis, but such use requires care, as liver damage may occur.

methoxamine. A sympathomimetic agent that increases the blood pressure by constriction of the peripheral vessels. It is used in the hypotension following spinal anaesthesia and postoperative shock. It has little cardiac or central stimulant action. Dose 10 to 15mg by i.v. or i.m. injection.

methoxyflurane. An inhalation anaesthetic of the halothane type, but with a less depressant action on the cardiovascular system. Usually given initially with nitrous oxide. It increases the action of muscle relaxants, which should be given in reduced doses. It has good analgesic properties, and is used with the Cardiff inhaler for intermittent analgesia in obstetrics. May cause liver damage, and should not be used as the sole anaesthetic agent, or in patients taking tetracycline

or any other nephrotoxic drug.

methoxyphenamine. A sympathomimetic agent with a selective bronchodilator action, and little cardiovascular activity. Used in bronchial and asthmatic patients as an alternative to related drugs. May cause some drowsiness. Dose 150 to 400mg daily.

Methrazone. Feprazone, *q.v.*

methyclothiazide. A diuretic similar to chlorothiazide, but with increased potency. Dose 2.5 to 10mg daily.

methyl cellulose. A derivative of cellulose that forms stable, mucilaginous solutions in water. Used as emulsifying agent and bulk laxative.

methylated spirit. Alcohol containing 5% of wood naphtha. Used for skin preparation and alcoholic applications. The methylated spirit used domestically is coloured violet to indicate its unsuitability for medicinal use.

methylcysteine. A sputum liquefier claimed to be of value in respiratory conditions where the sputum is viscid. Dose 600mg daily. May also be given by aerosol inhalation.

methyldopa. A potent hypotensive compound used in the treatment of hypertensive cardiovascular conditions. The drug produces a smooth reduction in blood pressure that is not significantly affected by exercise. The action is increased by the administration of thiazide diuretics. Drowsiness may occur during the early stages of treatment. Should be used with care in liver disease. Dose 0.5 to 2g daily.

methylphenidate. A central stimulant less powerful than the amphetamines, useful in narcolepsy and some psychiatric conditions. Dose 10mg.

methylphenobarbitone. A sedative with anticonvulsant properties. Given in epilepsy as an alternative to phenobarbitone, q.v. Dose as anticonvulsant 400 to 600mg daily.

methylprednisolone. A corticosteroid with the actions, uses and side-effects of prednisone, q.v.

methyltestosterone. An orally active form of testosterone, q.v. Tablets should be dissolved under the tongue for maximum absorption. Dose 5 to 50mg daily in divided doses.

methyprylone. A synthetic sedative and hypnotic with actions and uses similar to those of chloral, q.v. Dose 200 to 400mg.

methysergide. A synthetic drug related to ergometrine, but used empirically in the prophylaxis of migraine. Of no value in an acute attack. Dose 2 to 6mg daily.

Metilar. Paramethasone, q.v.

metoclopramide. An antiemetic of value in drug-induced nausea and vomiting. Of little use in travel sickness. Also used to induce gastric peristalsis during x-ray examination of the stomach. Dose 5 to 10mg.

metolazone. A diuretic similar to quinethazone q.v., but effective in doses of 5mg daily. Used mainly in hypertension, and combined therapy may permit a reduction in dose of other antihypertensive agents. Dose in oedematous states 5 to 20mg daily as a single dose.

metoprolol. A beta-blocking agent, q.v., mainly used in the control of angina, but also of value in hypertension. Dose in angina 50 to 100mg thrice daily, in hypertension doses up to 200mg twice daily may be required. Care is necessary in heart block, bradycardia and pulmonary disease. Occasionally given by slow i.v. injection in acute cardiac arrhythmias. Dose 1 to 2mg per minute up to a total of 10 to 15mg under strict supervision.

Metopyrone. Metyrapone, q.v.

Metosyn. Fluocinonide, q.v.

metronidazole. An orally effective drug for the treatment of vaginal and urethral trichomoniasis. Dose 200mg three times a day for seven days. Also used in acute intestinal amoebiasis in daily doses of 2.4g for five days. Of great value in the prophylaxis and treatment of infections caused by *anaerobic* pathogens, such as bacteroides, as well as some Gram-negative organisms. Often combined with gentamicin. Dose 400mg three times a day for seven days. Suppositories of 1g may be used as an alternative. In severe infections, doses of 500mg eight-hourly by intravenous infusion, replaced by oral therapy as soon as possible.

metyrapone. An inhibitor of glucocorticoid synthesis, and is used as a test of pituitary function. It also has an indirect diuretic action by reducing the formation of aldosterone, *q.v.*

mexenone. A benzophenone derivative that absorbs ultra-violet light. Used as a 2% cream for protection against sunburn.

mexiletine. An anti-arrhythmic drug that depresses excessive myocardial activity with little action on normal function. Used in the prophylaxis and control of ventricular arrhythmia. Initial dose 400 to 600mg, with maintenance doses of 200 to 250mg. Also given by intravenous infusion in doses of 200 to 250mg.

Mexitil. Mexiletine, *q.v.*

mezlocillin. An antibiotic with a wide range of activity that includes Gram-negative organisms such as *Pseudomonas* and *Proteus*. Useful in a wide range of systemic and local infections. In severe infections it is given by i.v. infusion in doses up to 25g daily; in less severe infections 8 to 16g daily. Doses of 1 to 2g can be given by deep i.m. injection. Lower doses are necessary in renal insufficiency. Penicillin hypersensitivity is a contra-indication.

mianserin. An antidepressant with reduced anticholinergic side-effects. Useful in all types of depression, including those where anxiety is also present. It should not be used with monoamine oxidase inhibitors, *q.v.*, or barbiturates. In epileptics, the dose of anticonvulsant may have to be increased. Dose 10mg twice a day, increased as needed to 30 to 60mg daily, or as a single dose at night.

miconazole. An antifungal agent used as a 2% cream in some fungal skin infections, and as pessaries (100mg) in vaginal candidiasis.

Midamor. Amiloride, *q.v.*

Milton. A stable solution of sodium hypochlorite with sodium chloride. Dilutions of 2.5 to 5% form useful antiseptic solutions.

Miltown. Meprobamate, *q.v.*

Minocin. Minocycline, *q.v.*

minocycline. A tetracycline derivative with the wide range of activity of the tetracycline antibiotics, but with a longer action. Dose 200mg initially, followed by 100mg twice daily.

Minodiab. Glipizide, *q.v.*

minoxidil. A peripheral vasodilator used with diuretics and antihypertensive agents in severe hypertension. Initial dose 5mg daily, slowly increased according to need to a maximum of 50mg daily. *Not* to be used alone, as salt retention, oedema and cardiac weakness may occur. Hypertrichosis is a frequent side-effect.

Mintezol. Thiabendazole, *q.v.*

mitobronitol. A cytotoxic agent with an action similar to that of busulphan, *q.v.*, and used mainly in chronic myeloid leukaemia. Dose 250mg daily until the white cell count falls, then 125mg daily according to need. May cause gastro-intestinal disturbances, alopecia and bone marrow depression, and haematological control is necessary.

Mitoxana. Ifosfamide, *q.v.*

Modecate. Fluphenazine, *q.v.*

Moditen. Fluphenazine, *q.v.*

Modrenal. Trilostane, *q.v.*

Mogadon. Nitrazepam, *q.v.*

Molipaxin. Trazodone, *q.v.*

Monistat. Miconazole, *q.v.*

monoamine oxidase inhibitors (MAOI). Monoamine oxidase is an enzyme concerned with the breakdown of serotonin, noradrenaline and adrenaline. Chemically, these substances are amines, and they are stored in many organs of the body, including the brain, where they function as transmitters of nerve impulses. The period for which they act is short, as they are rapidly metabolised by monoamine oxidase. An inhibition of the enzyme would permit an increase in the amount of these amines in the brain, and such an increase is associated with cerebral stimulation. On that basis, several enzyme inhibitors have been used in the treatment of depression, although the mode of action is probably far more complex than the simple one indicated above. These inhibitors have an extensive pharmacological action, and can increase the effects of pressor drugs, analgesics, anaesthetics, sedatives, CNS stimulants, and many other drugs. Even certain foods, particularly cheese, may cause a dangerous rise in blood pressure during MAOI therapy. Great care is necessary during combined therapy, and ideally 10 to 14 days should elapse after ceasing MAOI treatment before using other potent drugs. Examples of monoamine oxidase inhibitors are iproniazid (Marsilid), isocarboxazid (Marplan), phenelzine (Nardil) and tranylcypromine (Parnate).

monosulfiram. A useful parasiticide and fungicide. In scabies, a 25% solution is diluted two or three times with water, and applied after a bath to the whole body, except face and scalp. Also used as a 5% soap for prophylaxis and control in schools etc.

morphine. The principal alkaloid of opium. It is widely used for severe pain and the associated anxiety and stress, and in cardiac asthma, shock and blood loss. It also checks cough and reduces peristalsis, but may cause nausea and vomiting. Morphine is more active by injection than orally. It may increase an established respiratory depression, and that condition

is a contra-indication. Tolerance of the drug, and dangers of dependence, should be borne in mind if treatment is prolonged. Dose 8 to 20mg.

Motilium. Domperidone, *q.v.*

Motival. Fluphenazine, *q.v.*

Mucodyne. Carbocisteine, *q.v.*

mustine. An organic compound with cytostatic effects on growing cells similar to those produced by x-rays. It is used in Hodgkin's disease and other neoplastic conditions. Solutions, which must be freshly prepared, are given by slow intravenous infusion. Injection outside a vein causes very severe inflammation. Occasionally given by intrapleural injection in bronchial carcinoma. Average dose 5 to 8mg. Side-effects include nausea, alopecia, peptic ulcer and bone marrow depression. Close haematological control is necessary.

Myambutol. Ethambutol, *q.v.*

Mycardol. Pentaerythritol, *q.v.*

Mydriacyl. Tropicamide, *q.v.*

Mydrilate. Cyclopentolate, *q.v.*

Myelobromol. Mitobronitol, *q.v.*

Myleran, Busulphan, *q.v.*

Myocrisin. Sodium aurothiomalate, *q.v.*

Myodil. An oily iodine compound used in myelography.

Injected intrathecally in doses of 2 to 5ml.

Myotonine. Bethanechol, *q.v.*

Mysoline. Primidone, *q.v.*

N

Nacton. Poldine, *q.v.*

nadolol. A beta-blocking agent with the actions and uses of propranolol, *q.v.* Dose in angina 40mg daily, or more; dose in hypertension 80mg daily, increased slowly as required. Maximum daily dose 240mg.

naftidrofuryl. A peripheral and cerebral vasodilator. Claimed to be of value in cerebrovascular disorders, and to improve memory in the elderly. Dose 300 to 600mg daily; 40 to 80mg by i.m. injection daily; oral therapy continued for at least three months.

Nalcrom. Capsules of sodium cromoglycate, *q.v.*, for oral use as an adjunct in ulcerative colitis. Dose 800mg daily.

nalidixic acid. A synthetic antibacterial drug. Following oral administration, the blood levels are too low to be useful in systemic infections, but the drug is correspondingly of value in urinary infections, especially those due to Gram-negative organisms, except *Pseudomonas*.

Side-effects include nausea, drowsiness, dizziness, and rash. Care is necessary in renal and liver dysfunction. Dose 1g six-hourly.

naloxone. A powerful and rapidly acting antagonist of opiate narcotics, and quickly reverses the respiratory depression, coma and convulsions of opiate overdose. It is a specific antagonist of pentazocine, *q.v.* Dose 0.4 to 1.2mg i.v. Response to i.m. injection much slower. Repeated doses at intervals of 1 to 2 minutes may be given according to response. In children, initial doses of 5 to 10 micrograms i.v., but much larger doses may be necessary. Naloxone has also been used in septic shock.

nandrolone. A steroid derivative, related to testosterone, but with markedly reduced virilising properties. It has the anabolic or tissue-building properties of the parent compound, and is used in postoperative convalescence in both sexes. Also useful in osteoporosis and wasting diseases. Dose 25mg weekly by i.m. injection.

naphazoline. See Antistine-Privine.

Naprosyn. Naproxen, *q.v.*

naproxen. A non-steroidal anti-inflammatory agent useful as an alternative to other drugs in rheumatoid and similar conditions. Care is necessary in peptic ulcer. Dose 250mg twice a day.

Narcan. Naloxone, *q.v.*

Nardil. Phenelzine. *See* monoamine oxidase inhibitors.

Narphen. Phenazocine, *q.v.*

natamycin. An antifungal antibiotic used for candidiasis and trichomoniasis. Given as a suspension for oral candidiasis in infants (dose four drops after every feed); by aerosol inhalation in respiratory fungal infections; topically as a cream (2%). Used as vaginal tablets (25mg) in trichomoniasis.

Natrilix. Indapamide, *q.v.*

Natulan. Procarbazine, *q.v.*

Navidrex. Cyclopenthiazide, *q.v.* Navidrex-K contains potassium chloride in addition, to offset any potassium loss in the urine caused by the diuretic action of cyclopenthiazide.

Naxogen. Nimorazole, *q.v.*

Nebcin. Tobramycin, *q.v.*

nefopam. A powerful analgesic chemically unrelated to other analgesics. It causes little respiratory depression in standard doses. Useful in acute or chronic pain as an alternative to pethidine, *q.v.* Dose 30 to 90mg three times a day, or 20mg by injection.

Nefrolan. Clorexolone, *q.v.*

Negram. Nalidixic acid, *q.v.*

Nembutal. Pentobarbitone sodium, *q.v.*

Neo-Cytamen. Hydroxocobalamin, *q.v.*

Neo-Mercazole. Carbimazole, *q.v.*

neomycin. An antibiotic active against a wide range of organisms, but owing to its toxic nature when injected, it is used mainly in preparations for external use. It is often used together with hydrocortisone or other antiinflammatory steroid in the treatment of inflamed and infected areas, but prolonged use may cause allergy. Occasionally used as an intestinal antiseptic. Dose 2 to 8g daily.

Neo-Naclex. Bendrofluazide, *q.v.*

Neophryn. Phenylephrine, *q.v.*

Neoplatin. Cisplatin, *q.v.*

neostigmine. An inhibitor of cholinesterase which thus indirectly prolongs the action of acetylcholine released at nerve endings. Valuable in the treatment of myasthenia gravis in doses of 15 to 30mg. Widely used postoperatively to antagonise the residual effects of muscle relaxants of the tubocurarine and gallamine type in doses of 2.5 to 5mg i.v., after a preliminary injection of 0.5 to 1mg of atropine.

Nepenthe. A proprietary

preparation similar to tincture of opium.

Nephril. Polythiazide, *q.v.*

Nerisone. Diflucortolone, *q.v.*

Neulactil. Pericyazine, *q.v.*

niacin. Nicotinic acid, *q.v.*

niclosamide. A synthetic anthelmintic of value in the elimination of tapeworm. The drug is given fasting in a dose of 1g which is repeated in two hours, and followed by a purge. It has a toxic effect on the worm, which is killed by the drug; older remedies merely aided expulsion.

nicofuranose. A nicotinic acid derivative, *q.v.* It has an extended action of some value in peripheral vascular disorders. Dose 0.5 to 1g daily.

nicotinamide. A compound derived from nicotinic acid, *q.v.*, and possessing similar properties, but differs in that it has little vasodilator action. It is useful in deficiency states when the vasodilator action of nicotinic acid limits the dose.

nicotinic acid. An essential food factor, occurring in yeast, liver, etc, but now prepared synthetically. It is a specific in the treatment of pellagra. It causes vasodilation, and is used in Ménière's disease, chilblains, headache, angina pectoris. In very large doses it lowers the blood cholesterol level. Daily prophylactic dose 15 to 30mg. Daily therapeutic dose 50 to 250mg.

nicotinyl tartrate. This derivative has the vasodilator properties of nicotinic acid, *q.v.*, but they are less intense and the action is more prolonged. Useful in peripheral circulatory disturbances such as Raynaud's disease and acrocyanosis. Dose 100 to 200mg daily.

nicoumalone. A synthetic anticoagulant similar to phenindione, *q.v.* Initial dose 8 to 16mg; subsequent doses are based on the response, as shown by determination of the blood prothrombin levels.

nifedipine. A coronary vasodilator useful in angina pectoris. May cause flushing and headache. Dose 10 to 20mg three times a day.

nikethamide. A centrally acting respiratory stimulant with mild vasoconstrictor properties. Dose as injection of nikethamide (25%) 2 to 4ml by i.m. or i.v. injection.

Nilevar. Norethandrolone, *q.v.*

nimorazole. An orally active trichomonacide. For trichomoniasis in males and females, a single dose of 2g is given with the main meal; in Vincent's gingivitis 500mg twice a day for two days; in amoebiasis 500mg twice a day for five days. Contra-indicated in neurological disorders. Side-effects include nausea and drowsiness.

Nipride. Sodium nitroprusside, *q.v.*

niridazole. A schistosomicide valuable in some forms of infection with the blood fluke *Schistosoma*. The drug is metabolised in the liver, and should not be used in *S. japonicum* infections, where liver damage is common. It is also useful in amoebiasis and against guinea worm. Side-effects include nausea, anxiety and confusion. It should not be given to epileptics, and care is necessary in liver dysfunction. Dose 25mg per kg daily for five to seven days.

nitrazepam. A mild hypnotic of low toxicity that is of value in insomnia as an alternative to more toxic drugs. Even excessive overdose has few serious effects, but continuous use may have cumulative effects, and temazepam *q.v.*, is sometimes preferred when a shorter-acting drug is required. As with related drugs, the combined use with alcohol increases the central sedative action. Some nitrazepam-dependence has been reported. Dose 5 to 10mg.

nitrofurantoin. A urinary anti-septic with a wide range of activity. It is of value in renal infections that have become resistant to other forms of treatment. Average dose 100mg four times a day. Often used in rotation with other urinary antiseptics. Peripheral neuritis has occurred after extended treatment and in patients with renal impairment. Allergic reactions of the asthmatic type with pulmonary oedema have been reported, as have blood disorders and liver damage.

nitrofurazone. A wide-range antibacterial compound used mainly for infected wounds and preparation for skin grafting. Sensitisation may occur after continuous application. Occasionally used orally in the treatment of trypanosomiasis in doses of 1 to 2g daily.

nitrogen mustard. Mustine, *q.v.*

nitroglycerin. Glyceryl trinitrate, *q.v.*

nitrous oxide. The oldest inhalation anaesthetic. Supplied in blue cylinders, it is widely used for brief operative work, and for induction.

Nivaquine. Chloroquine, *q.v.*

Nivemycin. Neomycin, *q.v.*

Nizoral. Ketoconazole, *q.v.*

Nobrium. Medazepam, *q.v.*

Noludar. Methyprylone, *q.v.*

Nolvadex. Tamoxifen, *q.v.*

nomifensine. A well-tolerated antidepressant and anxiolytic agent. Has some CNS stimulant properties. May potentiate the action of other drugs in parkinsonism. Dose 75 to 200mg daily.

noradrenaline. The pressor hormone released at sympathetic nerve endings when such nerves are stimulated. It is also present with adrenaline in the medulla of the adrenal gland. It raises blood pressure mainly by a general vasoconstriction, whereas adrenaline increases the blood pressure by constricting the peripheral vessels and increasing the cardiac output. Given by slow intravenous infusion in the treatment of shock, peripheral failure, and low blood pressure states, but the response may fluctuate with small variations in dose. Dose 2 to 20 micrograms per minute, based on need and response. Great care must be taken to avoid extra-venous injection.

norethandrolone. A steroid related to testosterone, with similar tissue-building or anabolic properties, but with a markedly reduced virilising action. It can therefore be used for its protein-building properties in both sexes in convalescence, in wasting diseases, osteoporosis and senile debility. Use with care in liver dysfunction or prostate gland disturbances. Dose 10 to 20mg orally; 25mg by injection.

norethisterone. An orally active progestogen. Used in amenorrhoea and functional uterine bleeding. Dose 5 to 20mg daily. In lower doses in association with small doses of an oestrogen, norethisterone and related drugs are in wide use as oral contraceptives.

Norflex. Orphenadrine, *q.v.*

norgestrel. Also referred to as levonorgestrel. An orally active progesterone-like drug, and a powerful inhibitor of ovulation. Used as a constituent of mixed oral contraceptive products, and as a 'progestogen-only' oral contraceptive. Also used in association with oestrogens in menstrual disorders and endometriosis.

Normison. Temazepam, *q.v.*

Norpace. Disopyramide, *q.v.*

nortriptiline. A tricyclic antidepressant with actions, uses and side-effects similar to those of imipramine, *q.v.* May be used in association with a chlorpromazine-type drug if the depression is associated with anxiety and agitation. Dose 20 to 100mg daily.

Noxyflex. Noxythiolin, *q.v.*

noxythiolin. A urea derivative with antibacterial properties. Used as 1 to 2% solution for irrigation. For bladder instillation, the addition of a local anaesthetic is necessary.

Numotac. Isoetharine, *q.v.*

Nupercaine. Cinchocaine, *q.v.*

nux vomica. The seeds from which strychnine, *q.v.*, is obtained.

Nydrane. Beclamide, *q.v.*

Nystan. Nystatin, *q.v.*

nystatin. A fungicidal antibiotic, used in the prophylaxis and treatment of intestinal, vaginal and superficial candidiasis. Oral tablets contain 500000 units, pessaries contain 100000 units; cream and ointment 1%.

O

oestradiol. The oestrogenic hormone controlling ovulation and menstruation. Given in oestrogen deficiency, such as menopause, kraurosis, amenorrhoea, etc. Also used in malignant disease of the breast and prostate. Although active orally, it is usually given as oestradiol monobenzoate by i.m. injection in doses of 1 to 5mg. Some other derivatives of oestradiol have a much longer action, and oestradiol undecanoate is given in doses of 100mg every three weeks.

Omnopon. A preparation of opium alkaloids similar to papaveretum, *q.v.*

Oncovin. Vincristine, *q.v.*

One-Alpha. Alfacalcidol, *q.v.*

Operidine. Phenoperidine, *q.v.*

Opilon. Thymoxamine, *q.v.*

opium. The dried juice from the capsules of the opium poppy; a brown powder containing 10% of morphine. The action of opium is mainly that of its principal constituent, morphine, but the other alkaloids present modify the action, and opium is preferred to morphine, *q.v.*, when a constipating action is required, as in intestinal disorders. Opium preparations include tincture of opium or laudanum (dose 0.3 to 2ml); paregoric or camphorated tincture of opium (dose 2 to 4ml). Dose of opium 30 to 200mg.

Opren. Benoxaprofen, *q.v.*

Opticrom. A preparation of sodium cromoglycate, *q.v.*, used for vernal conjunctivitis.

Optimine. Azatadine, *q.v.*

Orabolin. Ethyloestrenol, *q.v.*

Oradexon. Dexamethasone, *q.v.*

Orap. Pimozide, *q.v.*

Orbenin. Cloxacillin, *q.v.*

orciprenaline. A bronchodilator similar to isoprenaline, *q.v.*

Orisulf. Sulphaphenazole, *q.v.*

orphenadrine. A spasmolytic drug, used in the treatment of parkinsonism, and for the relief of voluntary muscle spasm. Dose 200 to 400mg daily in divided doses.

Orthoxine. Methoxyphenamine, *q.v.*

Orudis. Ketoprofen, *q.v.*

Ospolot. Sulthiame, *q.v.*

ouabain (strophanthin-G). A cardiac drug similar to strophanthin-K, but twice as active. Dose 0.12 to 0.25mg as a single i.v. injection. See also strophanthus.

oxazepam. A minor tranquilliser with actions and uses similar to those of diazepam, *q.v.* Dose 45 to 180mg daily.

oxedrine. A pressor agent of the phenylephrine type, but less potent. Used in mild hypotension. Dose 100mg orally or by injection.

oxpentifylline. An aminophylline-like drug used mainly as a vasodilator in peripheral vascular disorders. Dose 600mg daily initially; maintenance doses 300mg daily. Also given by intravenous infusion in doses of 100mg daily, up to a maximum of 400mg daily.

oxprenolol. An adrenergic blocking agent similar in action and use to propranolol, *q.v.* Dose 40mg to 2g daily.

Oxycel. Oxidised cellulose in the form of woven gauze strips. Has haemostatic properties, and if left in a closed wound it is eventually absorbed.

oxycodone. A powerful narcotic analgesic with a prolonged action. Dose 5 to 20mg orally or by injection. Suppositories of 30mg may give night-long relief.

oxymetazoline. A long-acting nasal decongestant. Used as 0.05% drops twice a day.

oxymetholone. A steroid related to testosterone, and with similar anabolic or protein-building properties. In oxymetholone, and in related steroids, the anabolic action has been largely separated from the androgen or virilising action, thus permitting the use of this type of drug in female patients and children. Useful in metabolic disturbance after operation, in convalescence, osteoporosis and anorexia. Dose 5 to 30mg daily.

oxypertine. A tranquilliser used in anxiety neuroses, psychoses and withdrawn schizophrenic states. Dose 10 to 40mg in mild conditions, up to 300mg daily in schizophrenia. In higher doses it may cause nausea, dizziness and drowsiness.

oxyphenbutazone. A derivative

of phenylbutazone, with similar analgesic and anti-inflammatory properties. Also used locally as eye ointment. Dose 200 to 400mg daily, subsequently reduced as much as possible. Regular blood counts advisable. The drug should be discontinued if a favourable response does not occur in four to five days.

oxytetracycline. An antibiotic derived from cultures of *Streptomyces rimosus*. Has a very wide range of activity against many organisms, including some viruses, and is useful in penicillin-resistant conditions. Usually given orally, but i.m. and i.v. preparations are available. Intravenous injections must be given slowly in dilute solution to avoid thrombosis. Average adult dose 250mg six-hourly. Side-effects, including gastro-intestinal disturbances and rectal irritation, may occur if treatment is prolonged.

oxytocin. The oxytocic fraction of pituitary extract, *q.v.*, but also made synthetically. Used for the induction and maintenance of labour, and to control postpartum haemorrhage. Dose for induction and inertia of labour 1 to 5 units by intravenous infusion; doses of 2 to 5 units by i.m. or slow i.v. injection for postpartum haemorrhage. May be given orally as 'buccal' tablets, but the response is variable. Oxytocin nasal spray is used to stimulate lactation a few minutes before breast-feeding.

P

PAS. Sodium aminosalicylate, *q.v.*

P I D. Phenindione, *q.v.*

Pacitron. Tryptophan, *q.v.*

Palfium. Dextromoramide, *q.v.*

Paludrine. Proguanil, *q.v.*

Panadol. Paracetamol, *q.v.*

pancreatin. A preparation containing the pancreatic enzymes, trypsin, lipase and amylase. Used to aid digestion in pancreatic disease. Dose 0.5 to 1g.

pancuronium. A muscle relaxant similar to tubocurarine, *q.v.*, but with the advantage that it has little histamine-releasing or cardiovascular action. Dose 2 to 4mg i.v. initially, with 2mg supplements as required.

papaveretum. A preparation of the alkaloids of opium, containing approximately 50% of morphine. Used mainly by injection, often in association with hyoscine (scopolamine). Dose 10 to 20mg, orally or by injection.

papaverine. One of the

alkaloids of opium. It has little analgesic action, and is used mainly as a smooth muscle relaxant in peripheral vascular diseases, spasm and asthma. Dose 60 to 300mg orally, 30 to 100mg by injection. It has caused cardiac arrhythmias.

para-aminosalicylic acid. Sodium aminosalicylate, *q.v.*

paracetamol. A mild analgesic with few side-effects. It differs from aspirin in the absence of any anti-inflammatory action. Dose 0.5 to 1g.

Paradione. Paramethadione, *q.v.*

paraffin. A generic name for hydrocarbon mixtures. Soft paraffin is the common ointment base; liquid paraffin is a lubricant laxative. Hard paraffin is used in the wax bath treatment of rheumatic conditions.

paraformaldehyde. A solid form of formaldehyde; used mainly for disinfecting rooms, etc., by vapourisation.

paraldehyde. A colourless liquid with strong characteristic odour. It is a rapid-acting sedative similar in effect to chloral, but less depressant. It may be given orally as a mixture, or by i.m. injection. Occasionally given rectally after dilution with arachis oil. Dose 5 to 10ml orally, or by injection (using a *glass* syringe), 15 to 30ml rectally.

paramethadione. An anticonvulsant similar to troxidone, *q.v.*, and useful in petit mal that does not respond to that drug. Dose 900 to 1800mg daily.

paramethasone. A corticosteroid basically similar to prednisone, *q.v.*, but effective in doses of 4 to 12mg daily.

parathyroid. The small glands associated with the thyroid, controlling calcium metabolism. Damage or loss of function results in hypocalcaemic tetany, which can be relieved by calcium gluconate injections, followed by oral calciferol, *q.v.*, alfacalcidol, *q.v.*, calcitriol, *q.v.*, or dihydrotachysterol, *q.v.*

pargyline. A monoamine oxidase inhibitor used in the treatment of resistant hypertension. It also has mild, central stimulant properties, and may influence mood. Dose 10 to 25mg or more daily, according to response.

Parlodel. Bromocriptine, *q.v.*

Parnate. Tranylcypromine, *q.v.*

Parvolex. Acetylcysteine, *q.v.*

Pavulon. Pancuronium, *q.v.*

Peganone. Ethotoin, *q.v.*

pemoline. A central nervous

stimulant of medium potency. Useful in fatigue and reactive depression. Occasionally hallucinations may be a side-effect. Paradoxically, sometimes of value in hyperactive children. Dose 40 to 120mg daily.

Penbritin. Ampicillin, *q.v.*

penicillamine. A breakdown product of penicillin, which has the power of combining with certain metals to form a water-soluble, non-toxic complex that is excreted in the urine. It is used in Wilson's disease, which is due to the retention of copper in the body, and in poisoning by lead and mercury. Also used in rheumatoid arthritis no longer responding to other treatment but such use requires care. Toxic side-effects include nausea, alopecia, blood disorders, fever and allergic reactions. Dose 0.25 to 1.5g daily.

penicillin, benzyl penicillin, penicillin G. The first of the antibiotics, *q.v.* It is well tolerated and is widely used in the treatment of infections due to Gram-positive organisms and the spirochaetes of syphilis and yaws. It acts by preventing the development of the bacterial cell wall, but some groups of organisms vary widely in the degree of sensitivity. Penicillin is usually given by i.m. injection, and as it is rapidly excreted the action is relatively brief, but derivatives are available, such as procaine-penicillin, which have a longer action. Penicillin V is an orally active derivative. The dose of penicillin varies considerably according to need and response, but an average dose of soluble penicillin is 500 000 units; of procaine-penicillin 300 000 units; of penicillin V, 125 to 250mg. Methicillin, *q.v.*, cloxacillin, *q.v.* are derivatives of penicillin active against resistant *staphylococci*; ampicillin, *q.v.*, and amoxycillin, *q.v.*, are derivatives with a wide range of activity against Gram-positive and Gram-negative organisms; carbenicillin, *q.v.*, is active against *Pseudomonas aeruginosa*.

Penotrane. Pessaries containing hydrargaphen, *q.v.*

pentaerythritol. A tetranitrate derivative with properties resembling those of glyceryl trinitrate, *q.v.*, but with a more prolonged action. Used mainly in the prophylaxis of angina, as side-effects are relatively infrequent. Dose 10 to 30mg.

pentagastrin. A synthetic compound that resembles natural gastrin in its ability to stimulate gastric secretion. It is given by s.c. injection in doses of 6 micrograms per kg to test gastric secretory ability. It is less likely to cause the side-effects associated with the histamine test for gastric activity.

pentamidine. A synthetic drug used in early trypanosomiasis. Prophylactic dose 300mg i.m. Therapeutic dose 150 to 300mg i.m. daily for 7 to 15 days. When the CNS is involved, combined treatment with tryparsamide, *q.v.*, or melarsoprol, *q.v.*, is necessary. Also useful in *Pneumocystis carinii* infections in patients on immunosuppressive treatment.

pentazocine. A powerful analgesic of the morphine type, but free from addictive properties, although dependence may occur with long treatment. Side-effects include dizziness, nausea, headache, tachycardia and rash. Dose 25 to 100mg orally, every three to four hours, 30 to 60mg by injection.

Penthrane. Methoxyflurane, *q.v.*

pentobarbitone sodium. A short-acting barbiturate, given orally in doses of 100 to 200mg for insomnia. Doses of 250 to 500mg i.v. as an anticonvulsant.

peppermint oil. Aromatic carminative. Used as peppermint water as a flavouring agent in mixtures.

Peptavlon. Pentagastrin, *q.v.*

Pentovis. Quinestradol, *q.v.*

Percorten. Deoxycortone, *q.v.*

Pergonal. Menotrophin, *q.v.*

perhexiline. A vasodilator used in the prophylaxis of angina. Initial dose 100 to 200mg twice a day, reduced later as required, the full response may take one to two weeks to develop. Contra-indicated in severe renal and hepatic disease.

Periactin. Cyproheptadine, *q.v.*

pericyazine. A tranquilliser of the chlorpromazine type, used mainly in schizophrenia and severe anxiety states. Dose 10 to 25mg or more, according to need.

Peritrate. Pentaerythritol, *q.v.*

Peroidin. Potassium perchlorate, *q.v.*

perphenazine. A major tranquilliser with the actions, uses and side-effects of chlorpromazine, *q.v.*, but effective in lower doses. Psychiatric dose 8 to 24mg daily; anti-emetic dose 4 to 8mg.

Persantin. Dipyridamole, *q.v.*

Pertofran. Desipramine, *q.v.*

pethidine. A synthetic analgesic with spasmolytic properties.

Widely employed as an alternative to morphine for pre- and postoperative use. Of value in obstetrics as it has a less depressant action than morphine on the respiration. Dose 25 to 100mg orally, or by i.m. injection: 25 to 50mg or more by slow intravenous injection. Side-effects include dizziness, nausea and palpitations.

Pethilorfan. A mixture of pethidine, *q.v.* and levallorphan, *q.v.* It is claimed to reduce respiratory depression in obstetrics without loss of analgesic potency.

Pevaryl. Econazole, *q.v.*

Pexid. Perhexiline, *q.v.*

Phanodorm. Cyclobarbitone, *q.v.*

phenazocine. A synthetic morphine-like drug, with similar analgesic properties, but with a more rapid and longer action and effective in smaller doses. The side-effects are similar to those of morphine, *q.v.* Dose 5mg orally; 2 to 4mg by i.m. injection, 1 to 2mg i.v.

phenazopyridine. A urinary analgesic, useful in relieving the pain of cystitis and related conditions. Dose 300 to 600mg daily.

phenelzine. A monoamine oxidase inhibitor used in the treatment of depression. The action is not clear, but may be linked with a rise in the amount of noradrenaline and other amines in the brain. It has many side-effects, and care is necessary in liver and renal dysfunction, cardiovascular disease and epilepsy. The drug may potentiate the action of other drugs that act on the central nervous system. Dose 15 to 45mg daily.

Phenergan. Promethazine, *q.v.*

phenethicillin. A penicillin derivative that is effective orally, giving blood levels comparable with those following injections of penicillin. Indicated in infections due to penicillin-sensitive organisms, and in some resistant staphylococcal infections. Dose 125 to 500mg.

phenformin. An oral hypoglycaemic drug, unrelated to tolbutamide, and may be effective when tolbutamide has failed to lower the blood-sugar level. May also be given in association with other drugs. Side-effects include nausea and anorexia, but reports of lactic acidosis suggest care may be necessary. Dose 50 to 200mg daily.

phenindamine. An antihistamine of medium potency. It differs from most antihistamines in having a mild central stimulant action, and so rarely causes drowsiness. Dose 75 to 150mg daily.

phenindione. An oral anti-coagulant, with a reliable action. Initial dose 200 to 300mg, maintenance doses 25 to 100mg daily. May cause nausea and because of the risk of allergic reactions, it has been replaced by warfarin, *q.v.*

pheniramine. An antihistamine similar to, but less potent than chlorpheniramine. Dose 25 to 50mg.

phenobarbitone. A powerful sedative, hypnotic and anti-convulsant drug. It has the general properties of the barbiturates, and is also used in epilepsy, often with pheny-toin, *q.v.* Dose 30 to 125mg.

phenobarbitone sodium. The soluble form of phenobar-bitone, *q.v.*, having a more rapid action. Dose 30 to 125mg or more as a single dose by i.m. injection.

phenol. Once used as an anti-septic; present in Calamine Lotion for itching; occasion-ally injected intrathecally as 5% solution in glycerin for very severe pain in malig-nancy.

phenolphthalein. A white in-soluble powder, used as a purgative. It is often given with emulsion of liquid paraf-fin. Dose 50 to 300mg.

phenolsulphonphthalein. A red compound used by i.v. injec-tion in doses of 6mg as a test of renal function. In health, at least 50% of the test dose will be excreted in the urine one hour after the injection.

phenoperidine. A morphine-like analgesic, often used in association with droperidol, *q.v.* Dose 0.5 to 5mg by i.v. injection.

phenoxybenzamine. A periph-eral vasodilator, used in Raynaud's disease, vaso-spasm, and to control the hypertension caused by phaeochromocytoma. Dose 10 to 20mg by i.v. injection, increasing according to need and response.

phentolamine. An adrenolytic drug which can temporarily reverse the action of adrenaline and norad-renaline on the blood vessels. Used mainly in the diagnosis of phaeochromocytoma, and during surgical removal of the tumour. Dose 5 to 10mg, by i.v. or i.m. injection.

phenylbutazone. An anti-inflammatory analgesic used mainly in treatment of rheumatic and arthritic con-ditions. Relief of pain is usually rapid, although inflammatory swelling is reduced less quickly. Also useful in the treatment of gout. Gastric disturbance is not uncommon and mucosal ulceration, rash and blood disorders may occur. Blood counts during treatment are necessary. The dose should be reduced to a low maintenance level as soon as relief is obtained. Dose 200 to 400mg daily.

phenylephrine. A vasoconstrictor similar to adrenaline, but less toxic. Given in hypotensive states in doses of 1 to 5mg i.m. or 500 micrograms by slow intravenous injection. Sometimes valuable in paroxysmal auricular tachycardia. It is also used locally as 1:400 solution as nasal decongestive, and as eye drops, 0.1 to 10%

phenylmercuric nitrate. A mercurial antibacterial and antifungal agent. Once used in anti-fungal creams and as a preservative in injections.

phenytoin sodium. An anticonvulsant used in grand mal epilepsy. It has little hypnotic effect and combined treatment with phenobarbitone may evoke the best response. May cause skin rashes, dizziness, gastric disturbances, etc., and in a few cases marked overgrowth of gums. Dose 50 to 100mg thrice daily.

pholcodine. Closely resembles codeine in its selective depressant action on the cough centre, but it has no analgesic action. It is present in a range of products used for the relief of useless cough, and has the advantage over codeine of not causing constipation. Dose 5 to 15mg.

Phospholine. Ecothiopate, *q.v.*

phthalylsulphathiazole. A poorly absorbed sulphonamide occasionally used in gastro-intestinal infections, and for pre- and post-operative use in abdominal surgery. Dose 5 to 10g daily.

Physeptone. Methadone, *q.v.*

physostigmine. The alkaloid of calabar beans, used as miotic (0.25 to 1%) to counteract effects of atropine, and in the treatment of glaucoma. More irritant than pilocarpine, *q.v.* Solutions may turn pink on storage.

phytomenadione. Vitamin K_1. A natural form of vitamin K, *q.v.*, with a powerful and extended action. Given in haemorrhage of the newborn, dose 1mg i.v. or i.m. Also to the mother before delivery, dose 1 to 5mg i.m. Of value in severe haemorrhage caused by *oral* anticoagulants. Dose 5 to 20mg by slow i.v. or i.m. Also active orally, dose 5 to 20mg.

pilocarpine. Has the miotic action of physostigmine, *q.v.*, but the action is less intense, and of shorter duration. It has the advantage of being less irritant. Used in glaucoma as 0.5 to 4% solution.

Pimafucin. Natamycin, *q.v.*

pimozide. A tranquilliser of value in schizophrenia, as it reduces the delusions without causing drowsiness. Not effective in mania or hyperactivity. Dose 2 to 4mg initially as a single dose, increasing to 10mg daily.

pindolol. A beta-receptor blocking agent, *q.v.*, with actions and uses similar to those of propranolol, *q.v.* Less likely to cause bronchospasm. Dose 7.5 to 45mg daily.

piperacillin. A semi-synthetic penicillin of low toxicity and a wide range of activity that extends to *Pseudomonas* and anaerobes. It can be used in association with other antibiotics, and may be a first-choice drug in many life-threatening and multiple infections. Dose 2g intravenously three or four times a day, or 2g two or three times a day by intramuscular injection. Not active orally.

piperazine. An effective anthelmintic against threadworms and roundworms. Available as elixir and tablets. Dose 500mg twice a day (4 to 6 years), up to 1g twice a day (14 years and over).

Seven days' treatment is usually sufficient. Dizziness is a side-effect usually associated with higher doses. For roundworms a single dose of up to 4g is given according to age. The worms are narcotised, so a purge may be necessary to ensure expulsion before the effects of the drug disappear.

piperidolate. A weak atropine-like drug used mainly in gastro-intestinal spasm. Dose 200mg daily.

Pipril. Piperacillin, *q.v.*

Piriton. Chlorpheniramine, *q.v.*

piritramide. A powerful morphine-type analgesic used in the relief of postoperative pain. Not suitable for prolonged use as it may cause dependence. Dose 20mg by i.m. injection.

piroxicam. A powerful anti-inflammatory and analgesic agent. Of value in arthritis, spondylitis, gout and related conditions. Standard dose 20mg daily. In acute conditions, 40mg initially, and 20mg daily as necessary. As with related drugs, side-effects include gastro-intestinal disturbances of varying severity.

Pitocin. Oxytocin, *q.v.*

Pitressin. Vasopressin, *q.v.*

pituitary extract. An aqueous extract of the posterior lobe of the pituitary gland. Used chiefly by insufflation as an antidiuretic in diabetes insipidus. See also desmopressin.

pivampicillin. A more active derivative of ampicillin, with similar actions and uses. Is hydrolysed to ampicillin after absorption, but gives higher blood levels. Much is excreted in the urine, of value in urinary infections. Dose 350 to 700mg three or four times a day.

pivmecillinam. An orally-active form of mecillinam, *q.v.* Used mainly in urinary infections. Dose 200mg three or four times a day.

pizotifen. A serotonin antagonist used in the prophylaxis of migraine, and vascular headache. Dose 1.5 to 6mg daily.

podophyllum resin. A powerful purgative, but now used topically as a paint (5 to 25% in alcohol or liquid paraffin) for venereal and other warts. Very irritant on healthy tissues.

poldine. A synthetic atropine-like drug with a marked inhibitory action on gastric secretion. May cause dryness of the mouth. Used in hyperacidity and gastric ulcer. Dose 10 to 30mg daily.

polymyxin B. An antibiotic used in infections due to *Ps. aeruginosa* and other Gram-negative bacteria. Kidney damage and other toxic effects limit its systemic value and less toxic antibiotics such as carbenicillin, *q.v.*, and gentamicin, *q.v.*, are now preferred. Dose up to 25 000 units per kg daily by slow intravenous infusion. Also used for topical application, often in association with hydrocortisone.

polymyxin E. Colistin, *q.v.*

polythiazide. A potent diuretic with the actions, uses and side-effects of the thiazide diuretics but effective in the low dose of 1 to 4mg daily.

Ponderax. Fenfluramine, *q.v.*

Pondocillin. Pivampicillin, *q.v.*

Ponstan. Mefenamic acid, *q.v.*

potassium. One of the most important ions of the body, mainly present in intracellular fluid. Many diuretics increase loss of potassium as well as sodium; with extended treatment the potassium balance may be disturbed, with acute muscle weakness, cardiac arrhythmias, and an increased sensitivity to digitalis. Potassium loss can be treated with potassium chloride orally (often as Slow-K, but may cause peptic ulceration), or by effervescent potassium tablets. Mixed diuretic and potassium products are not entirely satisfactory. In acute potassium deficiency, various potassium-containing intravenous solutions are available, but dose and rate of administration require care, as in excess, potassium can cause cardiac arrest.

potassium citrate. A diuretic useful in cystitis and other inflammatory conditions of the urinary tract where the urine is acid; in gout, to increase the excretion of uric acid, and during sulphonamide therapy to prevent crystalluria. Dose 1 to 2g.

potassium iodide. It reduces the viscosity of bronchial mucus, and is used as an expectorant; it is of value in the prophylaxis and treatment of simple goitre which is due to a deficiency of iodide. Also given pre-operatively in thyrotoxicosis, as it alters the texture of the gland, and facilitates surgery. Dose as an expectorant 250 to 500mg, in thyrotoxicosis 150mg daily.

potassium perchlorate. Once used in thyrotoxicosis, as it indirectly influences the formation of thyroxine. Now rarely used therapeutically, as it may cause aplastic anaemia. Used occasionally in association with radioactive iodine as a test of thyroid activity.

potassium   permanganate. Purple crystals, soluble in water. A powerful oxidising and deodorising agent used 1:1000 as lotion, 1:10 000 to 1:5000   as   mouthwash, douche, bladder washout and bath.

povidone-iodine. A complex of iodine with an organic carrier such as povidone is termed an iodophore. When applied to the skin, iodophores slowly release iodine, and have an extended antiseptic action. Used for local application to the skin and mucous membranes as solution containing the equivalent of 0.75% to 1% of iodine.

Praxilene. Naftidrofuryl, *q.v.*

prazepam. A long-acting benzodiazepine with the general properties and side-effects of the benzodiazepines. Used for the symptomatic relief of anxiety and tension states. Dose 30mg daily. Repeated doses may lead to accumulation.

prazosin. A drug with a specific relaxant action on arteriolar smooth muscle. It produces a slow and sustained fall in blood pressure with few haemodynamic side-effects. Claimed to be of value in all grades of benign hypertension. Dose 2mg three times a day initially, adjusted after four to six weeks. Side-effects include dizziness, nausea, lethargy, oedema.

prednisolone. A derivative of hydrocortisone, with actions, uses and doses comparable with those of prednisone *q.v.*

prednisone. A derivative of cortisone, *q.v.*, with similar properties, but effective in lower dose, and causing less sodium retention and electrolyte disturbance. Prednisone and prednisolone are widely used in a variety of unrelated conditions, including arthritis, rheumatoid conditions, inflammatory skin conditions, in allergic states, and in status asthmaticus. Large doses are sometimes given in leukaemia and other blood disorders. Prednisone is also useful in nephrotic oedema. It is also used with other drugs as an immuno-suppressive agent in transplant surgery. Both prednisone and prednisolone may cause dyspepsia and peptic ulcer in susceptible patients, and for long-term suppressive treatment the dose should not exceed 8mg daily. For initial therapy and in crisis, the dose may vary from 20 to 100mg daily, adjusted to response as soon as the condition permits. Special products are available for i.m. and i.v. injection; for

intra-articular injection, and for local use as eye drops. Cortisone is preferred in adrenal deficiency states where a salt-retaining effect is essential.

Predsol, Prednesol. Brand names of some prednisolone products.

Pregnyl. Chorionic gonadotrophin, *q.v.*

prenylamine. A vasodilator used in the prophylactic treatment of angina. Dose 180 to 300mg daily.

Pressimmune. An equine immunoglobulin preparation obtained from horses by immunisation with human lymphocytes. It suppresses cell-mediated immunity, but has less influence on antibody production and resistance to bacterial infection. Used as an immunosuppressive agent in transplant surgery, after sensitivity tests, as allergic reactions are common.

Priadel. Lithium carbonate, *q.v.*

prilocaine. A local anaesthetic with the actions, uses and side-effects of lignocaine, *q.v.*

Primalan. Mequitazine, *q.v.*

primaquine. An anti-malarial drug of limited value, usually given in association with chloroquine for final treatment on return from malarial areas.

primidone. An anticonvulsant drug used in the treatment of grand mal and psycho-motor epilepsy, but some cases of petit mal also respond. The changeover from other forms of therapy should be gradual. Drowsiness is a not uncommon side-effect. Dose 250mg to 2g daily.

Primolut N. Norethisterone, *q.v.*

Primperan. Metoclopramide, *q.v.*

Pripsen. Granules containing piperazine, *q.v.*, and a senna extract, this providing an anthelmintic and a purge in a single dose of 10g.

Priscol. Tolazoline, *q.v.*

Pro-Banthine. Propantheline, *q.v.*

probenecid. An orally active compound that increases the excretion of uric acid, and so is useful in the treatment of gout. It is given in doses of 0.5 to 1g daily, together with alkalis. The drug also has the reverse property of delaying the excretion of penicillin and cephalexin and is given in doses of 0.5g six-hourly to raise the blood levels of those drugs.

procainamide. A procaine derivative occasionally of value in the treatment of cardiac arrhythmias. Dose 500mg orally or i.m., increased later to 1g. Intra-venous use in emergencies when a rapid response is essential requires care, as a marked fall in blood pressure may occur.

procaine hydrochloride. A local anaesthetic of the cocaine type, now largely replaced by lignocaine, *q.v.*

procaine penicillin. An old form of long-acting penicillin, given by i.m. injection in doses of 300 to 900mg daily. Resultant blood levels are low, so usually given together with penicillin G, *q.v.*, to obtain a higher initial blood level. Use best restricted to infections highly sensitive to penicillin.

procarbazine. A cytostatic agent that inhibits cell division. Useful in Hodgkin's disease and lymphomas that no longer respond to other drugs. Dose 50 to 300mg. Initial doses should be low to reduce nausea.

prochlorperazine. A major tranquilliser with the actions, uses and side-effects of chlorpromazine, *q.v.*, but is more powerful, and effective in lower doses. Anti-emetic dose 10 to 25mg. Psychiatric dose 15 to 100mg daily.

procyclidine. A spasmolytic drug similar to benzhexol, *q.v.*, used mainly in the treatment of parkinsonism.

Reduces rigidity more than tremor. Dose 7.5 to 30mg daily.

progesterone. The hormone of the corpus luteum, responsible for the preparation of the uterus to receive a fertilised ovum. Used occasionally in treatment of functional uterine haemorrhage. Dose 2 to 60mg by i.m. injection. Orally effective drugs such as dydrogesterone, *q.v.*, which have reduced oestrogenic and androgenic side-effects, are now preferred. Norethisterone, *q.v.*, is widely used in oral contraceptive products.

proguanil hydrochloride. A synthetic antimalarial of high potency and low toxicity, widely used in suppressive and therapeutic treatment. Dose 100 to 300mg daily.

Proladone. Oxycodone, *q.v.*

Proluton-Depot. Hydroxyprogesterone, *q.v.*

promazine. Has the actions, uses and side-effects of chlorpromazine, *q.v.* Useful in the treatment of restlessness in the aged. Dose ranges from 50 to 800mg daily, orally, i.v., or i.m.

promethazine. A long-acting antihistamine with sedative properties. Of value in urticaria, parkinsonism, and in premedication. Dose 20 to 50mg daily, orally or by i.m. injection, but the subsequent drowsiness may be undesirable.

Prominal. Methylphenobarbitone, *q.v.*

Prondol. Iprindole, *q.v.*

Pronestyl. Procainamide, *q.v.*

Propaderm. Skin preparation of beclomethasone, *q.v.*

propanidid. A short-acting intravenous anaesthetic, unrelated to the barbiturates. Recovery is rapid and complete, with few side-effects. Dose 5 to 10mg per kg body-weight as 5% solution.

propantheline. An atropine-like compound used as a spasmolytic in peptic ulcer, pylorospasm, ureteral spasms, etc. Side-effects include dryness of mouth and blurring of vision. Dose 45mg daily.

propranolol. A beta-adrenoceptor blocking agent, *q.v.*, that reduces the cardiac response to circulating adrenaline. It is of value in reducing the work load on the heart during exercise, and stress, and is used in the treatment of angina, coronary insufficiency, cardiac arrhythmias and hypertension. May cause bronchospasm in asthmatic patients. More cardio-selective drugs, such as acebutolol, *q.v.*, are now available. Dose 20 to 120mg or more daily, 3 to 10mg i.v.

propylthiouracil. A thyroid inhibitor occasionally used in thyrotoxicosis. Dose 50 to 200mg.

prostaglandin. A generic term applied to a series of closely related fatty acid derivatives, originally extracted from prostate gland, but now prepared synthetically. They are widely distributed in animal tissues, and have a complex and varying range of biological activity. Thus they may have a smooth muscle stimulating or relaxant action, pressor, vasodilator, inflammatory or other properties. There is evidence that the anti-inflammatory action of aspirin and related drugs may be due to an inhibition of prostaglandin synthesis. There are four main groups of prostaglandins (PGA, PGB, PGE and PGF) which can be further subdivided. PGE_2 and PGF_2 have been given by intravenous infusion in the induction of labour and in the termination of pregnancy, and an oral form is available as dinoprostone, q.v.

Prostigmin. Neostigmine, q.v.

Prostin E_2. Dinoprostone, q.v.

Prostin VR. A preparation of alprostadil (prostaglandin E_1) for intravenous use in maintaining the patency of the ductus arteriosus in neonates with congenital heart lesions requiring surgical correction. The temporary improvement in circulation so obtained permits improved diagnosis while surgery is considered. Dose 0.1 micrograms per kg per minute under strict control.

protamine sulphate. A simple protein obtained from fish sperm. It neutralises the anticoagulant effect of heparin, and it is used in controlling the haemorrhage that may occur during heparin therapy. It is given intravenously in doses of 5ml as a 1% solution; 1ml will neutralise about 1000 units of heparin.

Prothiaden. Dothiepin, q.v.

prothionamide. A tuberculostatic drug similar to ethionamide, q.v. Dose 0.75 to 1g daily. Useful when ethionamide is not tolerated.

protriptyline. A tricyclic antidepressant with a rapid action, and is largely free from any sedative properties. Similar to imipramine, q.v., in action, and if anxiety or tension is also present, it may be given with tranquillisers. Dose 15 to 60mg daily.

Provera. Medroxyprogesterone, q.v.

Pro-Viron. Mesterolone, q.v.

pseudoephedrine. A drug very

closely related to ephedrine, *q.v.*, but said to have reduced central effects. Used mainly as a respiratory decongestant. Adult dose 60 to 240mg daily, children 60 to 120mg daily.

Pularin. Heparin, *q.v.*

Pulmadil. Rimiterol, *q.v.*

Puri-Nethol. Mercaptopurine, *q.v.*

Pyopen. Carbenicillin, *q.v.*

pyrazinamide. A tuberculostatic drug used in infections resistant to standard treatment. Can be given alone for short periods, but for long treatment combined therapy is essential. May cause liver damage and hyperuricaemia. Dose 20 to 35mg per kg body-weight daily.

Pyridium. Phenazopyridine, *q.v.*

pyridostigmine. An anticholinesterase similar to neostigmine, *q.v.*, but with a slower and more prolonged action. Useful in myasthenia gravis and paralytic ileus. Dose 60 to 240mg orally, 1 to 5mg by i.m. injection.

pyridoxine (vitamin B_6). This vitamin plays an essential part in protein metabolism. Apart from deficiency states, it has been used in alcoholism, muscular dystrophy, agranulocytosis, nausea and vomiting of pregnancy. Dose 20 to 100mg.

pyrimethamine. An anti-malarial drug similar to proguanil, but its chief value is in prophylaxis. Regular use will inhibit most relapses of benign tertian malaria. Dose 25 to 50mg weekly. Also used with dapsone, *q.v.*, as Maloprim, *q.v.*, in chloroquine-resistant malaria.

Q

Questran. Cholestyramine, *q.v.*

quinalbarbitone sodium. A short-acting barbiturate. Used in mild insomnia and anxiety states. Dose 50 to 200mg.

quinestradol. An oestrogen with a relatively selective action on vaginal tissues. Used mainly in postmenopausal vaginitis. Dose 1 to 2mg daily.

quinethazone. A diuretic with the actions and uses of hydrochlorothiazide, *q.v.* Dose 50 to 100mg daily.

quinidine. An alkaloid of cinchona, similar to quinine, but it has a specific depressant effect on the atrial muscle. It has been used in the treatment of early atrial fibrillation and in paroxysmal tachycardia, but beta-adrenergic blocking agents, *q.v.*, are often preferred. Quinidine may cause tinnitus and other side-effects in sensitive patients, and a test dose of 200mg is often given. If tolerated, a dose of 300mg may be given three to five times a day. Treatment should be stopped if response does not occur within 10 days.

quinine. The principal alkaloid of cinchona bark. Dose 60 to 600mg. The old treatment for malaria. Now largely replaced by chloroquine, *q.v.*, and proguanil, *q.v.* Still of value in chloroquine-resistant falciparum malaria, and in severe conditions, quinine hydrochloride by i.v. injection may be life-saving.

R

ranitidine. A powerful histamine H_2 antagonist of the cimetidine, *q.v.*, type, but with a longer action. It reduces the volume, acidity and pepsin content of gastric secretion, and is of value in peptic ulcer, reflux oesophagitis and similar conditions. Dose 150mg morning and evening, continued for at least four weeks. Maintenance dose of 150mg at night. In severe conditions, ranitidine may be given by slow i.v. injection in doses of 50mg, repeated at intervals of six to eight hours. In sus-

pected gastric ulcer, malignancy should be excluded before treatment is commenced. Side-effects of this new drug have not yet been evaluated.

Rastinon. Tolbutamide, *q.v.*

Rauwiloid. A mixture of alkaloids of rauwolfia. The action is basically that of the main constituent, reserpine, *q.v.*

rauwolfia. The dried roots of *Rauwolfia serpentina*. Used in the treatment of hypertension because of its depressant action of the central nervous system. The action is mainly that of its chief alkaloid, reserpine, *q.v.* Dose 200mg daily initially, maintenance dose 50 to 300mg daily.

razoxane. A synthetic cytotoxic agent used in various sarcomas in combination with radiotherapy. Dose 125mg twice daily under laboratory control.

Razoxin. Razoxane, *q.v.*

Redeptin. Fluspirilene, *q.v.*

Redoxon. Ascorbic acid, *q.v.*

reserpine. The principal alkaloid of rauwolfia, *q.v.* It is used in mild hypertension, but a fall in blood pressure occurs only after continued treatment. Dose in hypertension 0.1 to 0.5mg daily. It may cause depression, nasal congestion and gastric disturbances, and more controllable drugs are now preferred.

Resonium A. An ion-exchange resin that takes up potassium and releases sodium. Used in some hyperkalaemic conditions, under biochemical control. Dose 15 to 30g three or four times a day. For a child 0.5 to 1g/kg daily.

resorcin. An antipruritic and keratolytic agent used mainly as ointment in acne, and as hair lotions for removing dandruff. Myxoedema has been reported following the prolonged use of resorcin preparations.

retinol. Vitamin A, *q.v.*

Rheomacrodex. A dextran, *q.v.*, preparation used mainly to improve blood flow and prevent 'sludging' of red cells after injury. Useful in various types of peripheral ischaemia.

Rheumox. Azapropazone, *q.v.*

rhubarb. The dried rhizome of various species of Rheum, from China and Tibet. Used occasionally as a mild purgative and in small doses as an astringent bitter.

riboflavine (vitamin B$_2$). An orange-yellow powder. It is part of the vitamin B complex, and is concerned with the oxidation of carbohydrates and amino-acids. A deficiency causes several characteristic effects, including angular stomatitis and 'burning feet'. It is given in doses of 1 to 10mg in deficiency states associated with restricted diets or poor absorption.

Rifadin. Rifampicin, *q.v.*

rifampicin. An antibiotic used with isoniazid, *q.v.*, in tubercular infections. It has largely replaced streptomycin, *q.v.* Dose 450 to 600mg daily before breakfast.

Rimactane. Rifampicin, *q.v.*

rimiterol. A drug basically similar to isoprenaline, *q.v.*, but with a more selective bronchodilator action. Given by aerosol inhalation in doses of 200 to 600 micrograms.

Ringer's solution. An electrolyte replacement solution containing sodium chloride, potassium chloride and calcium chloride.

Ritalin. Methyl phenidate, *q.v.*

ritodrine. A uterine relaxant of value in premature labour. Given initially by intravenous infusion in doses of 50 micrograms per minute. Later, oral therapy with doses of 10mg two- to six-hourly.

Rivotril. Clonazepam, *q.v.*

Robaxin. Methocarbamol, *q.v.*

Rocaltrol. Calcitriol, *q.v.*

Roccal. Benzalkonium, *q.v.*

Rogitine. Phentolamine, *q.v.*

Rondomycin. Methacycline, *q.v.*

Ronicol. Nicotinyl tartrate, *q.v.*

Ronyl. Pemoline, *q.v.*

rosoxacin. Acrosoxacin, *q.v.*

rutin. A glycoside obtained from buckwheat. It has been used in the treatment of capillary fragility. Dose 20mg. A related compound (Paroven) is used in vascular disorders of the legs in doses of 250mg three or four times a day.

Rynacrom. Sodium cromoglycate, *q.v.*

Rythmodan. Disopyramide, *q.v.*

S

saccharin. An organic chemical with a very sweet taste, widely used as a non-calorific substitute for sugar. Has been used by rapid i.v. injection (2.5g in 4ml) for arm-tongue circulation time.

Salazopyrin. Sulphasalazine, *q.v.*

salbutamol. A bronchodilator similar in action to isoprenaline, *q.v.*, but with a more selective action, and fewer cardiac side-effects. Dose 6 to 16mg daily.

salcatonin. Calcitonin, *q.v.*, obtained from salmon.

salicylic acid. Has useful keratolytic and fungicidal properties. Used as ointment (2%) for skin conditions, and as ointments and plasters (up to 40%) for corns and warts.

salsalate. A long-acting mild analgesic of the aspirin type, but less likely to cause any gastric disturbance. Dose 2 to 4g daily.

Saluric. Chlorothiazide, *q.v.*

Sanomigran. Pizotifen, *q.v.*

Saroten. Amitriptyline, *q.v.*

Saventrine. A long-acting form of isoprenaline, *q.v.*, used mainly in heart block. Dose 30mg.

Savlon. A mixture of cetrimide and chlorhexidine, *q.v.*, widely used as an effective and non-irritant antiseptic.

scopolamine. Hyoscine, *q.v.*

Seconal sodium. Quinalbarbitone sodium, *q.v.*

Sectral. Acebutolol, *q.v.*

Securopen. Azlocillin, *q.v.*

selenium sulphide. Used as a shampoo in the treatment of dandruff. Prolonged use may cause alopecia. Toxic orally.

Selexid. Mecillinam, *q.v.*, for oral use.

Selexidin. Mecillinam, *q.v.*, for injection.

Selora. Sodium-free salt substitute useful in salt-restricted diets.

Selsun. Selenium sulphide, *q.v.*

senna. The leaves and pods of *Cassia* sp., used as a purgative. Standardised preparations such as Senokot are now preferred.

Senokot. A proprietary preparation of senna from which undesirable constituents have been largely removed. Available as granules or tablets.

Septrin. Co-trimoxazole, *q.v.*

Serc. Betahistine, *q.v.*

Serenace. Haloperidol, *q.v.*

Serenid. Oxazepam, *q.v.*

serotonin. A substance present in many body cells, which may act as a neurotransmitter in the central nervous system. A reduction in brain serotonin levels may be associated with depression (see tryptophan). Some allergic reactions may also be linked with the action of serotonin on sensitised cells (see cyproheptadine).

Serpasil. Reserpine, *q.v.*

serum gonadotrophin. The follicle-stimulating hormone obtained from pregnant mares' serum. Used with oestrogens in amenorrhoea and functional uterine bleeding. Dose 200 to 1000 units by i.m. injection.

silver nitrate. Used mainly as silver nitrate sticks (caustic points) for cauterising warts. Once used as eye drops (1%) in the newborn, and still used for that purpose in the USA.

silver sulphadiazine. Sulphadiazine, *q.v.*, combined with silver. Used as a cream, 1% for burns and infected skin conditions where a prolonged action is required.

Effective against *Pseudomonas aeruginosa*.

Sinequan. Doxepin, *q.v.*

Sinthrome. Nicoumalone, *q.v.*

Sintisone. Prednisolone, *q.v.*

Slow-K. Tablets containing potassium chloride 600mg in a wax base from which the drug is slowly released in the gastro-intestinal tract. Used to offset the potassium loss that may occur during diuretic treatment.

soda-lime. A mixture of calcium and sodium hydroxides, used in closed-circuit anaesthetic apparatus to remove carbon dioxide.

sodium acetrizoate. An iodine compound used as a contrast agent in intravenous pyelography, etc. Available in strengths of 30%, 50% and 70%.

sodium acid phosphate. An acid diuretic, given with hexamine, *q.v.* In full doses it acts as a saline purgative. Dose 2 to 4g.

sodium aminosalicylate. This compound is exceptional in having a selective bacteriostatic action on the tubercle bacillus, yet it has no other antibacterial activity. It is widely used in the treatment of tuberculosis, as it is rapidly absorbed orally, but frequent dosing is necessary to maintain adequate blood levels. It must always be used with at least one other anti-tubercular drug such as rifampicin, *q.v.*, to avoid the development of drug-resistance. Dose 10 to 20g daily.

sodium aurothiomalate. A gold compound used in the treatment of active rheumatoid arthritis. It is of no value in other forms of the disease, or where bone change has already occurred. Given by intramuscular injection in doses of 10mg weekly initially, slowly increasing to 50mg weekly. The total dose during a course should not exceed 500mg. Side-effects are common, and may be severe. Contra-indicated in renal and hepatic disease, blood dys-crasia and hypertension.

sodium benzoate. When given by injection, it is excreted as hippuric acid, and the rate of excretion is sometimes used as an indication of liver function.

sodium bicarbonate. A widely used soluble antacid, often in association with less soluble antacids such as magnesium carbonate or trisilicate, *q.v.* Dose 1 to 4g. Of value by slow i.v. injection of an 8.4% solution in metabolic acidosis; weaker solutions usually given by i.v. infusion. Such weaker solutions of

value in forced alkaline diuresis.

sodium chloride. An important constituent of blood and tissues. Widely used by intravenous injection as normal saline (0.9%) or as dextrose saline in treatment of dehydration and shock. Its use as an emetic in the treatment of poisoning is no longer advised. Used externally as saline solution as a simple cleansing lotion.

sodium citrate. An alkaline diuretic similar to potassium citrate, *q.v.*, and given for similar purposes. Dose 1 to 4g. For citrating milk 100mg to each feed may be used.

sodium cromoglycate. A compound with a specific effect in blocking the action of histamine and other spas-mogens that cause broncho-spasm and asthma in sensit-ised patients. Used for the prophylactic treatment of allergic asthma by inhalation with a 'Spinhaler'. Dose 20mg. Also available together with isoprenaline. Special preparations are available for use in allergic rhinitis. Not absorbed orally, but may be useful as a sup-plementary drug in ulcerative colitis.

sodium edetate. A calcium chelating or binding agent occasionally used in hyper-

calcaemia. Given by intravenous infusion in a dose of
70mg/kg daily. A local
anaesthetic may be added to
reduce the pain of the injection. In severe hypercal-
caemia, larger doses have
been given, but may cause
renal damage. Also used locally as a 0.4% solution for
calcified corneal opacities.

sodium fusidate. An antibiotic
used mainly in staphylococcal infections resistant to
other drugs. Sometimes
given in association with
penicillin. Dose 500mg
eight-hourly with food. In
severe infections it may be
given by intravenous infusion.

sodium lactate. Has been used
as M/6 solution, or as Hartmann's solution, *q.v.*, by
intravenous infusion for
acidosis, but sodium bicarbonate, *q.v.*, is now preferred.

sodium nitroprusside. A short-
acting drug used in the control of hypertensive crisis,
and for controlled hypotension during anaesthesia.
Given by intravenous infusion as a 0.01% solution
under strict observation.

sodium perborate. White
powder soluble in water, with
antiseptic and deodorant
properties similar to hy-
drogen peroxide.

sodium picosulphate. A synthetic laxative similar to
bisacodyl, *q.v.*, but with a
slower action. Dose 5 to
15mg at night.

sodium salicylate. A soluble
analgesic and anti-
inflammatory agent. Used
mainly in acute rheumatic
fever in doses of 10g or more
daily. Such doses may cause
tinnitus and nausea. Other
side-effects are similar to
those of aspirin.

sodium sulphate. A saline purgative. Dose 2 to 15g. Also
used as a lotion (25%) to
promote drainage of infected
wounds.

sodium valproate. An anticonvulsant effective in most
forms of epilepsy. Adult dose
200mg twice daily initially,
increased as required to 800
to 1400mg daily. Side-effects
include nausea, drowsiness
and sometimes alopecia.

Soframycin. Framycetin, *q.v.*

Soneryl. Butobarbitone, *q.v.*

sorbide nitrate. Isosorbide dinitrate, *q.v.*

Sorbitrate. Isosorbide dinitrate, *q.v.*

Sotacor. Sotalol, *q.v.*

sotalol. A beta-adrenergic
blocking agent, *q.v.*, that is of
value in the treatment of
hypertension. It produces a
smooth reduction in blood
pressure, and the response is
not markedly influenced by

exercise. Dose 80mg initially, increasing as required to 240 to 600mg daily. A dose of 10 to 20mg may be given intravenously in cardiac arrhythmias. Care is necessary in heart block and bronchial disease, and in diabetes.

Sparine. Promazine, *q.v.*

spectinomycin. An antibiotic used in the treatment of gonorrhoea when penicillin is unsuitable. It is given by i.m. injection as a single dose of 2g for males and 4g for females. May cause nausea, dizziness and pruritus.

spironolactone. A diuretic that antagonises the action of aldosterone, *q.v.*, on the distal tubule. It increases the excretion of sodium, but reduces the excretion of potassium. Of value in oedema due to excessive secretion of aldosterone, *q.v.* May be given with other diuretics in hepatic cirrhosis. Side-effects include drowsiness and impotence. Dose 100 to 200mg daily.

Stadol. Butorphanol, *q.v.*

stanozolol. An anabolic steroid with actions and uses similar to those of nandrolone, *q.v.* Dose 5mg daily.

starch. Carbohydrate granules obtained from maize, rice, wheat or potato. Widely used as absorbent dusting powder.

Stelazine. Trifluoperazine, *q.v.*

Stemetil. Prochlorperazine, *q.v.*

stibophen. A complex antimony compound, less toxic than tartar emetic, *q.v.* Used for schistosomiasis as injection of stibophen (6.4%), i.m. or i.v. Dose 300mg on alternate days to a total of 2.4 to 4.5g.

stilboestrol. A synthetic oestrogen, active orally, and of value in menopausal conditions and for the suppression of lactation. Dose 0.1 to 5mg. It is also useful in the treatment of prostatic carcinoma, when very large doses may be required. Fosfesterol, *q.v.*, has a more intense and localised effect in such carcinomas.

streptokinase-streptodornase. A mixture of enzymes obtained from haemolytic streptococci. It has the property of liquefying purulent exudates, blood clots, etc., and is used to clean foul wounds, pressure sores, ulcers, etc. Streptokinase has been given intravenously in the early treatment of some thrombo-embolic disorders, often in association with hydrocortisone.

streptomycin. An antibiotic obtained from *Streptomyces griseus*. Occasionally used in urinary infections, and with penicillin in mixed infections. It is mainly used in tuberculosis, although rifampicin, *q.v.*, is now frequently preferred. Drug resistance may develop rapidly, so in tuberculosis combined treatment with isoniazid, *q.v.*, and other drugs is essential. High doses can cause permanent deafness. Cutaneous sensitisation may follow contact of the drug with the skin. Occasionally given by mouth in intestinal infections. Dose up to 1g daily by i.m. injection; up to 100mg by intrathecal injection; up to 1g six-hourly orally.

Stromba. Stanozolol, *q.v.*

strophanthus. Has cardiac properties similar to digitalis. Used mainly by i.v. injection as strophanthin-K or as ouabain, *q.v.*

strychnine. The alkaloid of nux vomica, *q.v.* It has a very bitter taste and it is used occasionally as gastric tonic, but has no other therapeutic value. Dose as Tincture of Nux Vomica, 0.6 to 2ml.

Stugeron. Cinnarizine, *q.v.*

Sublimaze. Fentanyl, *q.v.*

succinylsulphathiazole. A poorly-absorbed sulphonamide used in gastrointestinal infections, and for pre- and postoperative use in abdominal surgery. Dose 10 to 20g daily.

sulfadoxine. A long-acting sulphonamide, used mainly with pyrimethamine, *q.v.*, in resistant and falciparum malaria. Prophylactic dose 500mg with pyrimethamine 25mg; therapeutic dose, a single, double or treble dose, not to be repeated for at least seven days.

sulfametopyrazine. A long-acting drug with the general antibacterial properties of the sulphonamides, *q.v.* Dose 2g once a week.

sulindac. An anti-inflammatory and analgesic drug of value in arthritic and related conditions. May cause gastrointestinal disturbances and bleeding, and its use requires care. Dose up to 400mg daily.

sulphacetamide. A sulphonamide used as sulphacetamide soluble eye drops (10 to 30%) and an ointment (2.5 to 10%).

sulphadiazine. One of the more active and less toxic sulphonamides, *q.v.*; effective against streptococci, meningococci and many other organisms. Initial dose 3g, followed by 1 to 1.5g four-hourly. Given intravenously as sulphadiazine sodium in severe infections such as meningococcal meningitis.

sulphadimethoxine. A long-acting sulphonamide, *q.v.*, effective in a wide range of infections due to sulphon-amide-sensitive organisms, especially staphylococci. Dose 1 to 2g initially, followed by 0.5g daily.

sulphadimidine. One of the least toxic of the sulphonamides. Crystalluria and renal complications are rare, and the drug is particularly suitable for children. Initial dose 3g; followed by six-hourly maintenance doses of 1.5g. Smaller maintenance doses of 1g may be adequate in urinary infections. Sulphadimidine soluble is suitable for i.v. or deep i.m. injection.

sulphafurazole. A sulphonamide of particular value in urinary infections. Initial dose 3g followed by 1 to 1.5g, four- or six-hourly.

sulphaguanidine. A sulphonamide now largely replaced by phthalyl- and succinyl-sulphathiazole, *q.v.*

sulphamerazine. A sulphonamide resembling sulphadiazine in activity, but the slower excretion increases the risk of crystalluria. It is rarely given alone, but survives in mixed products such as Sulphatriad, *q.v.*

sulphamethizole. A sulphonamide used in the treatment of urinary infections. The low dose is exceptional, being 100 to 200mg,

five to seven times a day, and side-effects are uncommon.

sulphamethoxazole. A long-acting sulphonamide used mainly in urinary and respiratory infections. Dose 2g initially, followed by 1g twice daily. Adequate fluid intake during treatment is necessary to reduce side-effects.

sulphamethoxypyridazine. A long-acting sulphonamide, used mainly for prophylaxis or the treatment of chronic urinary or systemic infections. Dose 1g initially, then 0.5g daily. The slow elimination may complicate the treatment of side-effects.

Sulphamezathine. Sulphadimidine, *q.v.*

sulphanilamide. One of the earliest 'sulpha' drugs. Now replaced by more active compounds.

sulphaphenazole. A readily absorbed but slowly excreted sulphonamide, *q.v.* Dose 1g every 12 hours initially, then 500mg 12-hourly for three days.

sulphapyridine. A sulphonamide occasionally used for dermatitis herpetiformis not responding to dapsone, *q.v.*

sulphasalazine. A sulphonamide which is said to be taken up selectively by the connective tissue of the intestines. Useful in the treatment of chronic ulcerative colitis. Dose 1g, four to six times a day.

sulphathiazole. One of the early sulphonamides. Occasionally used in mixed products such as Sulphatriad, *q.v.*

Sulphatriad. Tablets of sulphadiazine, sulphathiazole and sulphamerazine. A mixture of sulphonamides is considered to reduce the overall toxic effects. Initial dose 4 tablets, then 2 tablets four-hourly.

sulphinpyrazone. A drug related to phenylbutazone, but with the selective action of increasing the excretion of uric acid, hence used in the treatment of chronic gout. Dose 200 to 400mg daily. The drug also increases blood platelet survival time, and is now used in the post-treatment of myocardial infarction. It is given in doses of 800mg daily, starting about one month after the attack. Prolonged treatment may be necessary.

sulphonamides. A group of drugs that has an antibacterial action by preventing the uptake and use of folic acid, which is essential for cell nutrition. They are thus bacteriostatic and not bactericidal in action. The members of the group differ mainly in the rate of absorption and excretion, and in frequency of dose. Side-effects include nausea and dyspepsia, diarrhoea and allergic reactions. Bone marrow damage may occur if treatment is prolonged. The rare Stevens-Johnson syndrome is a serious reaction. Sulphadimidine, *q.v.*, is a widely used drug of this group.

sulphur. Greenish-yellow insoluble powder once used as ointment for scabies; present in many products of alleged value in acne. It has been used as a laxative. Dose 1 to 4g.

sulthiame. An anticonvulsant of use in most epileptic conditions except petit mal. It is usually given in association with other anticonvulsants. Dose 200 to 600mg daily.

suramin. A complex organic chemical used in the treatment of the early stages of trypanosomiasis; of no value in later stages as it does not enter the cerebrospinal fluid. Dose 1g, i.v. at weekly intervals for five weeks, after an initial dose of 200mg to test tolerance.

Surmontil. Trimipramine, *q.v.*

Suscardia. Isoprenaline, *q.v.*

Sustac. A long-acting preparation of glyceryl trinitrate, *q.v.*

suxamethonium. A short-acting muscle relaxant, with an

action lasting three to five minutes. A preliminary injection of an intravenous barbiturate must be given, as the first effect of suxamethonium is to cause painful muscle contraction before the relaxant action supervenes. Dose 20 to 100mg i.v.; further doses according to need, or by infusion of a 0.1 to 0.2% solution.

Symmetrel. Amantadine, *q.v.*

Sympatol. Oxedrine, *q.v.*

Synacthen. Tetracosactrin, *q.v.*

Synadrin. Prenylamine, *q.v.*

Synalar. Fluocinolone, *q.v.*

Synkavit. Menadiol, *q.v.*

Syntocinon. Synthetic form of oxytocin, *q.v.*

Syntopressin. Synthetic form of vasopressin, *q.v.* Used as nasal spray in the treatment of diabetes mellitus.

T

Tace. Chlorotrianisene, *q.v.*

Tacitin. Benzoctamine, *q.v.*

Tagamet. Cimetidine, *q.v.*

talampicillin. A derivative of ampicillin, *q.v.*, with similar therapeutic applications. High blood levels are obtained with standard doses of 250mg three times daily.

talc. A soft white form of magnesium silicate, extensively used as dusting powder. It is also used as lubricant for surgeons' gloves but may cause a talc granuloma if it gains access to the tissues during operations, and glove powders prepared from starch are now preferred.

Talpen. Talampicillin, *q.v.*

tamoxifen. A synthetic compound with anti-oestrogenic but not androgenic properties. This selective action is unusual, and the drug is free from the side-effects of androgens used as anti-oestrogens. Of value in the post-menopausal treatment of breast cancer. Dose 10mg twice daily.

Tanderil. Oxyphenbutazone, *q.v.*

tannic acid. An astringent obtained from oak galls. It is an antidote in acute alkaloid poisoning, and is used as suppositories for its astringent effects in haemorrhoids.

Taractan. Chlorprothixene, *q.v.*

tartar emetic. Antimony and potassium tartrate, *q.v.*

Tavegil. Clemastine, *q.v.*

Tegretol. Carbamazepine, *q.v.*

Telepaque. Iopanoic acid, *q.v.*

temazepam. A mild hypnotic of the nitrazepam, *q.v.*, type, but with a shorter duration of action. Often useful in the elderly. Dose 10 to 30mg, increased if necessary to 60mg.

Temgesic. Buprenorphine, *q.v.*

Temetex. Diflucortolone, *q.v.*

Tenormin. Atenolol, *q.v.*

Tensilon. Edrophonium, *q.v.*

Tenuate. Diethylpropion, *q.v.*

terbutaline. A bronchodilator similar in action and uses to salbutamol, *q.v.* Useful in bronchospasm due to allergic or intrinsic asthma.

terfenadine. An antihistamine with reduced sedative side-effects. Of general value in hay fever and allergic skin conditions. Dose 60mg twice a day.

Teronac. Mazindol, *q.v.*

Terramycin. Oxytetracycline, *q.v.*

Tertroxin. Liothyronine, *q.v.*

testosterone. The androgenic hormone of the testes, which controls the development of the male sex characteristics. Used in male underdevelopment, and gynaecomastia. In the female it is sometimes used to control uterine bleeding, and in large doses is of value in the palliative treatment of certain forms of carcinoma of the breast. Usually given by i.m. injections as testosterone propionate, but special tablets (100mg) for implantation in the tissues for a prolonged action are available. Dose 25 to 100mg i.m. and 100 to 600mg by implantation.

Tetmosol. Monosulfiram, *q.v.*

tetrachloroethylene. An anthelmintic used against hookworms. Dose 3 to 5ml as a single dose, repeated after four to seven days. Side-effects include nausea, headache. Care necessary in liver or kidney damage.

tetracosactrin. A synthetic form of the active part of corticotrophin, *q.v.*, with similar actions and uses. Of value in patients allergic or unresponsive to natural corticotrophin. 1mg i.v. is equivalent to 100 units of corticotrophin. Long-acting forms for i.m. injection are given in doses of 1mg at intervals of one to three days. Useful in single dose of 0.25mg as diagnostic test of adrenal cortex function, as cortisol level should normally rise within an hour.

tetracycline. A wide-range antibiotic very similar both chemically and pharmacologically to chlortetracycline, oxytetracycline, clomocycline and related compounds referred to generically as the tetracyclines. They all have the same type of action against both Gram-positive and Gram-negative organisms, but exhibit certain differences in solubility, absorption and excretion. These differences are reflected in the different doses, as tetracycline is given in doses of 250mg four times a day, whereas with doxycycline a single daily dose of 100mg may be adequate. Long treatment with a tetracycline may lead to gastro-intestinal disturbance owing to changes in the normal bacterial population of the intestinal tract.

Tetracyn. Tetracycline, *q.v.*

Tetralysal. Lymecycline, *q.v.*

Thalazole. Phthalylsulphathiazole, *q.v.*

theobromine. A weak diuretic related to theophylline, *q.v.* It survives in some mixed products used in hypertension.

theophylline. A bronchodilator with the actions and uses of aminophylline, *q.v.* Its use is increasing as long-acting forms, and a syrup for children, have become available. Dose 60 to 200mg up to four times a day. Proportionate doses for children.

Thephorin. Phenindamine, *q.v.*

thiabendazole. An anthelmintic effective against a wide range of intestinal parasites. Also useful in creeping eruption. Dose 50mg/kg daily, up to a maximum of 3g for one to three days.

thiacetazone. An antitubercular drug used with other drugs to prevent resistance. Initial dose 12.5 to 25mg, increased up to 200mg daily. Numerous side-effects limit its value.

thiambutosine. Used in the treatment of leprosy, as it may have a more rapid initial effect than dapsone, *q.v.* Resistance may occur after prolonged treatment. Dose 500mg to 2g daily. Sometimes given by injection in doses of 200mg to 1g weekly.

thiamine. Also known as aneurine and vitamin B_1. It is essential for carbohydrate metabolism, but is used clinically mainly in cases of deficiency, as in beri-beri, or when the diet is restricted. Also of value in the neuritis of pregnancy and alcoholism. Prophylactic dose 2 to 5mg daily; therapeutic dose 25 to 100mg daily.

Thiazamide. Sulphathiazole, *q.v.*

thiethylperazine. Although related to chlorpromazine, this drug is used only as an anti-emetic, as it has no significant tranquillising action. Dose 10 to 30mg daily orally, or by i.m. injection.

thioguanine. An antineoplastic agent similar in action and uses to mercaptopurine, *q.v.* Dose 2mg/kg daily.

thiomersal. A mercurial antiseptic and fungicide.

thiopentone. A widely used short-acting barbiturate given by intravenous injection for basal narcosis or anaesthesia. Solutions should be freshly prepared. Dose 100 to 500mg. Great care must be taken to avoid injection outside a vein, as the solution is very alkaline, and may cause necrosis.

thiopropazate. A tranquilliser similar in action to chlorpromazine, *q.v.* Useful in agitated and aggressive psychotic patients. Dose 15 to 30mg daily.

thioridazine. A tranquillising drug related to chlorpromazine, and used in similar doses for the treatment of various psychiatric conditions. Unlike most related drugs, it has no anti-emetic properties. Dose 30 to 600mg daily.

thiotepa. A cytotoxic drug similar in action to mustine, *q.v.*, but not irritant. Used in a variety of cancerous conditions, usually by i.v. injection in doses of 15 to 30mg, repeated according to the response. Larger doses have been injected directly into tumours.

thymoxamine. A peripheral vasodilator that is useful in a wide range of peripheral ischaemic conditions. Dose 60 to 480mg daily orally, 5 to 20mg daily by i.v. injection.

thyroid. The dried gland of the ox, sheep or pig from which thyroxine, *q.v.*, is obtained.

Thyroid gland is now rarely prescribed, as thyroxine, *q.v.*, is preferred, as absorption is more reliable, and the response more consistent.

thyroxine. The active constituent of thyroid, *q.v.*, but also prepared synthetically. Thyroxine is a powerful metabolic stimulant, specific in cretinism, myxoedema and thyroid deficiency generally. In cretinism, early diagnosis and treatment is essential for full recovery, and therapy is life-long. In other deficiency states, initial doses should be small, and increased slowly. Rapid treatment or overdose may cause tachycardia, insomnia and diarrhoea. Dose 0.05 to 0.2mg daily.

Ticar. Ticarcillin, *q.v.*

ticarcillin. An antibiotic with actions and uses very similar to those of carbenicillin, *q.v.* In some cases the activity is increased by the additional use of aminoglycoside antibiotics such as gentamicin, which should be injected separately. Dose up to 24g daily by i.m. or i.v. injection.

timolol. A beta-adrenergic blocking agent of the propranolol (*q.v.*) type, used in the control of angina and hypertension. Care is necessary in bradycardia, cardiac insufficiency and bronchial disease. Dose 5mg thrice daily initially, slowly adjusted to maintenance dose of 15 to 45mg daily. It is also of value as eye drops (0.25% to 0.5%) in simple chronic glaucoma, as it reduces intra-ocular pressure by reducing the formation of the aqueous humour.

Timoptol. Timolol, *q.v.*

Tinaderm. Tolnaftate, *q.v.*

tobramycin. An antibiotic of the gentamicin type, but more active against *Ps. aeruginosa*. Often has an increased action when given with carbenicillin, *q.v.* Also useful in Gram-negative infections generally. Given by i.m. injection or intravenous infusion in doses of 3 to 5mg/kg daily. Care is necessary to avoid the ototoxic and nephrotoxic effects of this type of drug.

tocopherol. Also known as vitamin E. Has been given in habitual abortion, in some muscle disorders, and a variety of other conditions. Proof of its value is lacking. Dose 10 to 50mg daily.

tofenacin. A mild antidepressant of value in the elderly. Use with care in glaucoma or prostatic hypertrophy. Dose up to 80mg three times a day.

Tofranil. Imipramine, *q.v.*

Tolanase. Tolazamide, *q.v.*

tolazamide. An oral hypoglycaemic drug related to tolbutamide, *q.v.* Used in late-onset diabetes in doses of 100 to 200mg daily.

tolazoline. A peripheral vasodilator, exerting its greatest effects on the small vessels of the extremities. It is given in Raynaud's disease and similar conditions; and is used occasionally as drops in keratitis, iritis, etc. Dose 50 to 200mg daily.

tolbutamide. A sulphonyl derivative of urea similar to chlorpropamide, *q.v.*, and of value in diabetes. It is effective orally, and appears to act by stimulating the pancreas to produce or release more insulin, as it is effective only when some part of the pancreas is still active. It thus functions as an 'insulin sparer' and not as a substitute. The best results are obtained with middle-aged and mild diabetics normally stabilised on low doses of insulin. Juvenile and severe diabetics are not suitable cases for tolbutamide therapy. Dose, after stabilisation, 1 to 3 tablets daily (0.5 to 1.5g). A return to insulin may be necessary during illness.

Tolectin. Tolmetin, *q.v.*

tolmetin. An anti-inflammatory-analgesic agent used in rheumatoid and musculo-skeletal conditions. As with related drugs, it may cause gastro-intestinal disturbances in some patients, and should be taken after food. Hypersensitivity reactions may occur occasionally. Dose 0.6 to 1.8g daily.

tolnaftate. A synthetic anti-fungal agent used topically in tinea and other fungal infections of the skin.

Torecan. Thiethylperazine, *q.v.*

Trancopal. Chlormezanone, *q.v.*

Trandate. Labetolol, *q.v.*

tranexamic acid. An anti-fibrinolytic agent similar to amino-caproic acid, *q.v.* Used in local and general fibrinolytic conditions. Dose up to 4.5g daily, or up to 3g daily by i.v. injection.

Tranxene. Clorazepate, *q.v.*

tranylcypromine. A mono-amine oxidase inhibitor, *q.v.*, of use in severe depression not responding to other drugs. Dose 20mg daily initially, increased to 30mg daily or more according to need.

Trasicor. Oxprenolol, *q.v.*

Trasylol. Aprotinin, *q.v.*

trazodone. An antidepressant chemically distinct from other drugs, and with no anti-cholinergic side-effects. For all types of depression. Also has some anxiety-reducing properties. Response may be slow, and drowsiness a side-

effect. Dose 50mg twice or three times a day, increased if necessary to a maximum of 600mg daily.

Tremonil. Methixene, *q.v.*

Trescatyl. Ethionamide, *q.v.*

Trevintix. Prothionamide, *q.v.*

triamcinolone. One of the steroids of the cortisone type, but differs from the older drug in being more effective in lower dose, and with fewer side-effects. Useful in all conditions requiring cortisone therapy, except adrenal deficiency states, as it has no salt-retaining properties. Dose 4 to 48mg daily initially, reduced later to a maintenance dose of 8mg daily or less. Used locally as triamcinolone acetonide in inflamed skin conditions.

triamterene. A powerful diuretic, unrelated to the thiazides, and often effective in conditions not responding to those drugs. Triamterene acts mainly on the distal renal tubule, whereas the thiazides act on the proximal tubule. In severe oedematous conditions triamterene and a thiazide diuretic may be given together. Dytide is a mixture of triamterene and benzthiazide for such use. Dose 150 to 250mg daily.

triazolam. An hypnotic of the nitrazepam, *q.v.*, type, but effective in much smaller doses. Suitable for elderly patients, as an extended response is unlikely. It has caused psychological disturbances in some patients. Dose 125 to 250 micrograms.

trichloroacetic acid. Deliquescent crystals, used as a powerful caustic for warts.

trichloroethylene. A liquid similar to chloroform and used occasionally as an inhalation anaesthetic. It should not be used in closed-circuit anaesthetic apparatus owing to the formation of toxic breakdown products. The drug also has some analgesic properties and small doses inhaled from crushable glass ampoules are useful in trigeminal neuralgia.

triclofos. A derivative of chloral, *q.v.*, with the sedative properties of the parent drug, but is less irritant to the gastric mucosa. It can therefore be presented as tablets. Dose 0.5 to 1g.

Tridil. Glyceryl trinitrate, *q.v.*, prepared for intravenous infusion in the treatment of refractory angina, and in myocardial ischaemia.

Tridione. Troxidone, *q.v.*

trifluoperazine. A tranquillising drug of the chlorpromazine type, but with reduced sedative and increased stimulant properties. Also useful as an anti-emetic. Used in a wide range of mental conditions including psychosis, schizophrenia, hallucinations, and in lower doses for emotional states, nausea, etc. Dose 1 to 25mg according to need.

trifluperidol. A powerful tranquilliser of the haloperidol (*q.v.*) type, used chiefly in the control of mania and schizophrenia. May cause extrapyramidal side-effects, and care is necessary in liver dysfunction. Dose 1 to 8mg daily according to need.

Trilene. Trichloroethylene, *q.v.*

trilostane. An inhibitor of enzyme system concerned with production of mineralo- and glucocorticosteroids. Used to control adrenal cortex hyperfunction in hypercorticolism and related conditions. Close control essential. Pregnancy must be excluded. Dose 60mg four times a day initially, increased according to response.

Triludan. Terfenadine, *q.v.*

trimeprazine. A phenothiazine derivative with greater anti-allergic and anti-emetic potency than promethazine or chlorpromazine. Valuable in pruritus and many other itching conditions, in premedication, in some psychiatric conditions, and as a sedative for children. Dose 10 to 40mg daily.

trimetaphan. A short-acting ganglionic blocking agent. It is used to produce a controllable reduction in blood pressure during neuro- and vascular surgery when a relatively bloodless field is necessary. It is given by slow intravenous infusion, the dose being governed by the response, which varies very considerably. Frequent determination of blood pressure during use is essential.

trimethoprim. An antimalarial drug similar to pyrimethamine, *q.v.* It also has an antibacterial action by inhibiting bacterial folate enzymes, and is used in the prophylaxis and suppression of urinary tract and respiratory infections due to sensitive bacteria. Dose 300mg daily at night or 200mg twice a day. Lower doses in renal insufficiency. When given in association with a sulphonamide, the activity is increased and the risk of bacterial resistance is reduced. That synergistic action is the basis of products such as Septrin, Bactrim and Coptin.

trimipramine. An antidepressant drug similar to imipramine, *q.v.* Useful when the response to related drugs is inadequate. Dose 25 to 150mg daily according to need and response.

Triperidol. Trifluperidol, *q.v.*

triprolidine. A long-acting antihistamine, with an effect that persists over 12 hours. Suitable for children in appropriate doses, when given as a syrup. Dose 5 to 7.5mg daily.

trisodium edetate. Sodium edetate, *q.v.*

Trobicin. Spectinomycin, *q.v.*

tropicamide. A mydriatic and cycloplegic agent similar to homatropine, *q.v.*, but said to have a more rapid and shorter action. Used as 0.5% and 1% solution.

troxidone. An anticonvulsant used in petit mal epilepsy. It may cause some toxic effects, including skin rashes, and photophobia. Less common reactions include agranulocytosis and aplastic anaemia, and regular blood counts are essential. Initial doses should be small, and increased slowly according to need and response. Dose 0.3 to 2g daily.

tryparsamide. Used in late trypanosomiasis when the CNS is involved. Dose 1 to 3g by injection weekly, up to a maximum of 24g. May damage optic nerve, and melarsoprol, *q.v.*, is often preferred.

trypsin. A proteolytic enzyme of the pancreas. Highly purified fractions are used by local application for their proteolytic effects, or given by injection in thrombosis and inflammatory conditions.

Tryptizol. Amitriptyline, *q.v.*

tryptophan. An amino-acid present in the diet, that is the precursor of serotonin, *q.v.* A deficiency of serotonin in the brain is associated with some forms of depression, and the administration of tryptophan increases the brain level of serotonin. The response is slow, and some months of treatment is necessary before any relief of depression can be assessed. Dose 1g three times a day initially, doubled later if required.

Tubarine. Tubocurarine, *q.v.*

tuberculin. Concentrated filtrate of cultures of *Mycobacterium tuberculosis*. Used in the diagnosis of tuberculosis as Mantoux test.

tubocurarine. The muscle relaxing constituent of curare. Used in conjunction with general anaesthetics to increase relaxation during surgery; in the treatment of tetanus, and in the convulsive or shock treatment of mental disorders. Patients with hepatic impairment may be relatively resistant. The effects of tubocurarine are increased by ether and some other substances. The effects can be terminated by the injection of atropine and neostigmine, *q.v.* Dose 10 to 15mg i.v., followed by additional doses if required of 2 to 4mg at intervals of 25 minutes to a total of 45mg.

tyloxapol. A surface-active agent used by inhalation to liquefy thick bronchial secretions.

tyrothricin. A mixture of antibiotics derived from cultures of *Bacillus brevis*. Contains gramicidin, *q.v.* Used mainly as lozenges for mouth infections, or as a cream or lotion for burns and skin infections.

U

Ubretid. Distigmine, *q.v.*

Ukidan. Urokinase, *q.v.*

Ultandren. Fluoxymesterone, *q.v.*

Ultralanum. Fluocortolone, *q.v.*

undecenoic acid. Has useful antimycotic properties. It is used mainly as powder or ointment (5%), often with zinc undecylenate in the treatment of athlete's foot and associated conditions.

urea. Given intravenously as a 30% solution to reduce cerebral oedema following injury. Has been given orally as a diuretic in doses of 5 to 15g. A single dose of 15g is sometimes given to test renal function. Applied locally as a 10% solution, it promotes granulation and reduces odour from foul ulcers.

Ureaphil. A preparation of urea, *q.v.*, for intravenous infusion.

Urispas. Flavoxate, *q.v.*

urokinase. A plasmin activator obtained from human male urine. Valuable as a fibrinolytic agent in thrombosis, and in the solution of blood clots in the eye. Given by i.v. infusion in doses of 4000 units/kg hourly as required. For blood clots in the eye, a dose of 25 000 units is injected into the chamber. Also useful for clearing blocked AV shunts.

Urolucosil. Sulphamethizole, *q.v.*

ursodeoxycholic acid. Used for the dissolution of cholesterol gallstones. Dose 300mg twice a day for some months.

Uticillin. Carfecillin, *q.v.*

Uvistat. Menexone, *q.v.*

V

vaccines. Bacterial vaccines are suspensions or extracts of dead bacteria. They may be given by s.c. or i.m. injection, and are used mainly for prophylaxis against a particular infection. The most commonly used vaccines include anti-typhoid-para-typhoid vaccine (TAB), cholera vaccine, and whooping-cough vaccine. Smallpox vaccine and yellow fever vaccine are prepared from the corresponding viruses.

Valium. Diazepam, *q.v.*

Vallergan. Trimeprazine, *q.v.*

Valoid. Cyclizine, *q.v.*

Vancocin. Vancomycin, *q.v.*

vancomycin. An antibiotic used in overwhelming staphylococcal infections resistant to other antibiotics. Dose 2g daily by slow i.v. injection. Also used orally in staphylococcal enteritis and pseudomembranous colitis. Dose 2g daily.

Varidase. Preparation of streptokinase, *q.v.* and streptodornase.

Vascardin. Isosorbide dinitrate, *q.v.*

vasopressin. A preparation of the blood-pressure-raising and antidiuretic factors of the pituitary gland. It has been used in doses of 0.5 to 0.75ml in diabetes insipidus, but has been largely superseded by desmopressin *q.v.*

Vasoxine. Methoxamine, *q.v.*

Vatensol. Guanoclor, *q.v.*

Veganin. Tablets of aspirin, paracetamol and codeine.

Velbe. Vinblastine, *q.v.*

Velosef. Cephradine, *q.v.*

Ventolin. Salbutamol, *q.v.*

verapamil. Decreases the oxygen demands of the heart, and is used in the prophylaxis and treatment of angina. Dose 120 to 420mg daily.

Veriloid. Preparations of alkaloids of green hellebore. Occasionally used in hypertension. Dose 2 to 12mg daily.

Vermox. Mebendazole, *q.v.*

Vibramycin. Doxycycline, *q.v.*

vidarabine. An antiviral agent used as ointment 3% in herpes kerato-conjunctivitis. Also used by slow intravenous infusion with care for chickenpox and varicella zoster in patients receiving immunosuppressive therapy. Dose 10mg/kg daily for at least five days. May cause gastro-intestinal and haematological disturbances.

viloxazine. An antidepressant without sedative effects. Useful in mixed anxiety-repressive states, and in depression in epileptics. May increase the action of phenytoin and antihypertensive agents. Dose 150 to 300mg daily.

vinblastine. An alkaloid of periwinkle that has cytotoxic properties. Used chiefly in Hodgkin's disease and lung cancer. Dose 0.1mg per kg body-weight weekly by i.v. injection, increasing by 0.05mg weekly until adequate response.

vincristine. An alkaloid of periwinkle, used in the treatment of leukaemia in children. Dose 30 to 50 micrograms per kg body-weight weekly by i.v. injection.

vindesine. An alkaloid related to vinblastine, *q.v.* It has myelosuppressive properties, and is used in myeloid and lymphatic leukaemia and malignant melanoma. Dose is based on skin area; given intravenously under haematological control.

Vira-A. Vidarabine, *q.v.*

Visclair. Methylcysteine, *q.v.*

Visken. Pindolol, *q.v.*

vitamin A. One of the vitamins obtained from fish-liver oils. A deficiency in the diet causes night-blindness, skin changes and a decreased resistance to infection. Dose 2500 to 25 000 units daily.

vitamin B. A group of water-soluble vitamins obtained from yeast or rice polishings. The constituents include thiamine, *q.v.*, riboflavine, nicotinic acid, pyridoxine, and small amounts of other factors.

vitamin B$_6$. Pyridoxine, *q.v.*

vitamin B$_{12}$. Cyanocobalamin, *q.v.*

vitamin C. Ascorbic acid, *q.v.*

vitamin D. The vitamin essential for the absorption of calcium and phosphorus and subsequent bone formation. Several forms of the vitamin are known, but it is used chiefly as calciferol, *q.v.* Vitamin D is activated in the liver and kidneys to more powerful derivatives such as calcitriol, *q.v.*, and alfacalcidol, *q.v.*

vitamin D$_2$. Calciferol, *q.v.*

vitamin E. The vitamin present in wheat-germ oil, now largely replaced by the synthetic form tocopherol, *q.v.*

vitamin K. The vitamin concerned with the formation of prothrombin, and so with blood coagulation. Given as menadiol, *q.v.*, in haemorrhagic disorders. Of no value when the prothrombin level of the blood is adequate. Vitamin K$_1$, or phytomenadione, *q.v.*, has a similar but more rapid and sustained action.

Vivalan. Viloxazine, *q.v.*

Voltarol. Diclofenac, *q.v.*

W

warfarin. A synthetic anticoagulant similar to phenindione, *q.v.*, but with reduced side-effects. It is effective in lower doses, and tablets of 1, 3, 5 and 10mg are available. Dose is based on the prothrombin level, and is determined on individual requirements.

Welldorm. Dichloralphenazone, *q.v.*

Whitfield's ointment. Benzoic acid 6%, salicylic acid 3%. Has keratolytic and fungicidal properties, and is used mainly for ringworm.

wool alcohols. A water-in-oil emulsifying agent obtained from wool fat. It is used in many water-containing ointments, such as ointment of wool alcohols and hydrous ointment.

X

xipamide. A long-acting diuretic and antihypertensive similar to chlorthalidone, *q.v.* In hypertension, 20mg is given as a morning dose; in oedematous states, 40 to 80mg as a single morning dose, reduced later as necessary.

Xylocaine. Lignocaine, *q.v.*

Y

yeast. The fungus used in the fermentation of sugars to produce alcohol. Dried yeast has been used as dietary supplement for its vitamin B content.

Yomesan. Niclosamide, *q.v.*

Yutopar. Ritodrine, *q.v.*

Z

Zaditen. Ketotifen, *q.v.*

Zantac. Ranitidine, *q.v.*

Zarontin. Ethosuximide, *q.v.*

Zelmid. Zimelidine, *q.v.*

zimelidine. An antidepressant that selectively enhances transmission in serotonin neural systems. It has little anticholinergic action, and is useful in some major depressive states. Dose 200mg daily.

Zinacef. Cefuroxime, *q.v.*

Zinamide. Pyrazinamide, *q.v.*

zinc oxide. Soft white powder widely used in dusting powders, ointments, pastes, etc., for its mild astringent and antiseptic properties. Constituent of Lassar's paste, Unna's paste, calamine lotion and similar preparations.

zinc peroxide. Insoluble white powder with an antiseptic action similar to hydrogen peroxide but slower and more prolonged. Used as lotion (40%), mouthwash (25%), ointment (20%).

zinc stearate. A white insoluble powder used as a mild astringent in dusting powders for eczema and associated conditions.

zinc sulphate. Used as an astringent and stimulating lotion for indolent ulcers; and in conjunctivitis. Small doses (220mg) with meals are stated to promote healing of wounds.

zinc undecenoate. White insoluble powder. Constituent of dusting powders and ointments for mycotic conditions.

Zomax. Zomepirac, *q.v.*

zomepirac. An analgesic-anti-inflammatory agent used in arthritic and rheumatoid conditions, and musculo-skeletal pain. Contraindicated in peptic ulcer, or hyper-sensitivity to related non-steroidal agents. Dose 100mg six-hourly, up to a maximum of 600mg daily.

Zovirax. Acyclovir, *q.v.*

Zyloric. Allopurinol, *q.v.*

Approved and Proprietary Names of Drugs

APPROVED AND PROPRIETARY NAMES OF DRUGS

New drugs are usually introduced under a brand or proprietary name, but in many cases 'Approved' or non-proprietary names are also in use. The following lists give both the Approved Name and Proprietary Name of a number of available drugs. It does not include mixed products.

Approved Name	Proprietary Name	Main Action, Type of Drug or Use
acebutolol	Sectral	beta-adrenoceptor blockade
acepifylline	Etophylate	spasmolytic
acetazolamide	Diamox	glaucoma
acetohexamide	Dimelor	oral hypoglycaemic
acetylcysteine	Airbron;	mucolytic;
	Parvolex	paracetamol overdose
acrosoxacin	Eradacin	gonorrhoea
actinomycin D	Cosmegen	antineoplastic
acyclovir	Zovirax	antiviral agent
alcuronium	Alloferin	muscle relaxant
alfacalcidol	One-Alpha	vitamin D deficiency
allopurinol	Zyloric; Caplenal	uricosuric
allyloestrenol	Gestanin	progestogen
aloxiprin	Palaprin	antirheumatic
amantadine	Symmetrel	parkinsonism
ambenonium	Mytelase	myasthenia gravis
amikacin	Amikin	antibiotic
amiloride	Midamor	diuretic
aminocaproic acid	Epsikapron	haemostatic

amiodarone	Cordarone X	anti-arrhythmic
amitriptyline	Saroten; Tryptizol	antidepressant
amoxycillin	Amoxil	antibiotic
amphotericin	Fungizone; Fungilin	antifungal antibiotic
ampicillin	Penbritin; Amfipen; Pentrexyl	antibiotic
ancrod	Arvin	anticoagulant
aprotinin	Trasylol	enzyme inhibitor
atenolol	Tenormin	hypertension
azapropazone	Rheumox	antirheumatic
azatadine	Optimine	antihistamine
azathioprine	Imuran	antimetabolite; immunosuppressive
azlocillin	Securopen	antibiotic
bacampicillin	Ambaxin	antibiotic
baclofen	Lioresal	muscle relaxant
bamethan	Vasculit	vasodilator
beclamide	Nydrane	anticonvulsant
beclomethasone	Becotide; Propaderm	corticosteroid
bemegride	Megimide	respiratory stimulant
bendrofluazide	Aprinox; NeoNaclex	diuretic
benorylate	Benoral	antirheumatic
benoxaprofen	Opren	antirheumatic
benperidol	Anquil	tranquilliser
benzalkonium chloride	Roccal	antiseptic
benzathine penicillin	Penidural	antibiotic
benzhexol	Artane	parkinsonism

137

Approved Name	Proprietary Name	Main Action, Type of Drug or Use
benzoctamine	Tacitin	tranquilliser
benztropine	Cogentin	parkinsonism
bephenium hydroxynaphthoate	Alcopar	anthelmintic
betahistine	Serc	Ménière's disease
betamethasone	Betnelan; Betnovate	corticosteroid
bethanechol	Myotonine	smooth muscle stimulant
bethanidine	Esbatal	antihypertensive
biperiden	Akineton	parkinsonism
bisacodyl	Dulcolax	laxative
bretylium tosylate	Bretylate	anti-arrhythmic
bromhexine	Bisolvon	mucolytic
bromocriptine	Parlodel	anti-lactation; acromegaly
brompheniramine	Dimotane	antihistamine
bumetanide	Burinex	diuretic
bupivacaine	Marcain	anaesthetic
buprenorphine	Temgesic	analgesic
busulphan	Myleran	antineoplastic
butorphanol	Stadol	analgesic
butriptyline	Evadyne	antidepressant
calcitonin	Calcitare	hormone
calcitriol	Rocaltrol	vitamin D deficiency
candicidin	Candeptin	antimycotic
capreomycin	Capastat	antibiotic
captopril	Capoten	severe hypertension
carbamazepine	Tegretol	anticonvulsant; analgesic

138

carbaryl	Carylderm; Derbac	parasiticide
carbenicillin	Pyopen	antibiotic
carbenoxolone	Biogastrone; Duogastrone	peptic ulcer
carbimazole	Neo-Mercazole	thyrotoxicosis
carbocisteine	Mucodyne	mucolytic
carfecillin	Utilcillin	antibiotic
carisoprodol	Carisoma	muscle relaxant
carmustine	BICNU	antineoplastic
cefaclor	Distaclor	antibiotic
cefamandole	Kefadol	antibiotic
cefotaxime	Claforan	antibiotic
cefoxitin	Mefoxin	antibiotic
cefuroxime	Zinacef	antibiotic
cephalexin	Ceporex; Keflex	antibiotic
cephaloridine	Ceporin	antibiotic
cephalothin	Keflin	antibiotic
cephazolin	Kefzol	antibiotic
cephradine	Velosef	antibiotic
chenodeoxycholic acid	Chendol	gallstone solvent
chlorambucil	Leukeran	antineoplastic
chloramphenicol	Chloromycetin	antibiotic
chlordiazepoxide	Librium	tranquilliser
chlorhexidine	Hibitane	antiseptic
chlormethiazole	Heminevrin	soporific
chlormezanone	Trancopal	tranquilliser
chloroquine	Nivaquine; Avloclor	antimalarial
chlorothiazide	Saluric	diuretic

139

Approved Name	Proprietary Name	Main Action, Type of Drug or Use
chlorotrianisene	Tace	oestrogen
chlorpheniramine	Priton	antihistamine
chlorpromazine	Largactil	tranquilliser
chlorpropamide	Diabinese; Melitase	oral hypoglycaemic
chlorprothixene	Taractan	tranquilliser
chlortetracycline	Aureomycin	antibiotic
chlorthalidone	Hygroton	diuretic
cholestyramine	Questran	bile acid sequestrant
choline theophyllinate	Choledyl	bronchodilator
ciclacillin	Calthor	antibiotic
cimetidine	Tagamet	peptic ulcer
cinchocaine	Nupercaine	anaesthetic
cinnarizine	Stugeron	anti-emetic
cinoxacin	Cinobac	antibiotic
cisplatin	Neoplatin	antineoplastic
clemastine	Tavegil	antihistamine
clindamycin	Dalacin C	antibiotic
clobazam	Frisium	tranquilliser
clobetasol	Dermovate	corticosteroid
clobetasone	Eumovate	corticosteroid
clofazimine	Lamprene	antileprotic
clofibrate	Atromid-S	hypercholesterolaemia
clomiphene	Clomid; Serophene	infertility
clomipramine	Anafranil	antidepressant
clomocycline	Megaclor	antibiotic

clonazepam	Rivotril	anticonvulsant
clonidine	Catapres; Dixarit	antihypertensive, migraine
clopamide	Brinaldix	diuretic
clopenthixol	Clopixol	schizophrenia
clorazepate	Tranxene	tranquilliser
clorexolone	Nefrolan	diuretic
clotrimazole	Canestan	antimycotic
cloxacillin	Orbenin	antibiotic
colistin	Colomycin	antibiotic
corticotrophin	Acthar	hormone
cortisone	Cortelan; Cortisyl	corticosteroid
crotamiton	Eurax	antipruritic
cyanocobalamin	Cytacon; Cytamen	anti-anaemic
cyclandelate	Cyclospasmol	vasodilator
cyclizine	Marzine; Valoid	anti-emetic
cyclobarbitone	Phanodorm	hypnotic
cyclofenil	Rehibin	infertility
cyclopenthiazide	Navidrex	diuretic
cyclopentolate	Mydrilate	mydriatic
cyclophosphamide	Endoxana	antineoplastic
cyproheptadine	Periactin	antihistamine
cyproterone	Androcur	anti-androgen
cytarabine	Cytosar	antineoplastic
dacarbazine	DTIC	antineoplastic
danazol	Danol	pituitary suppressant
danthron	Dorbanex	laxative
dantrolene	Dantrium	muscle relaxant

141

Approved Name	Proprietary Name	Main Action, Type of Drug or Use
debrisoquine	Declinax	antihypertensive
demecarium bromide	Tosmilen	glaucoma
demeclocycline	Ledermycin	antibiotic
deoxycortone	Percorten M	Addison's disease
deserpidine	Harmonyl	antihypertensive
desferrioxamine	Desferal	iron poisoning
desipramine	Pertofran	antidepressant
deslanoside	Cedilanid	cardiac stimulant
desmopressin	DDAVP	diabetes insipidus
dexamethasone	Decadron; Dexacortisyl; Oradexon	corticosteroid
dexamphetamine	Dexedrine	appetite depressant
dextran	Dextraven; Lomodex; Rheomacrodex	plasma substitute
dextromoramide	Palfium	analgesic
dextropropoxyphene	Doloxene	analgesic
diazepam	Valium; Atensine	tranquilliser: muscle relaxant
diazoxide	Eudemine	antihypertensive; hypoglycaemia
dichloralphenazone	Welldorm	hypnotic
dichlorphenamide	Daranide; Oratrol	glaucoma
diclofenac	Voltarol	antirheumatic
dicyclomine	Merbentyl	antispasmodic
diethylcarbamazine	Banocide	filaricide
diethylpropion	Tenuate	appetite depressant
diflucortolone	Nerisone	corticosteroid

142

diflunisal	Dolobid	analgesic
digoxin	Lanoxin	cardiac failure
dihydrocodeine	DF 118	analgesic
dihydroergotamine	Dihydergot	migraine
dihydrotachysterol	AT 10; Tachyrol	hypocalcaemia
dimenhydrinate	Dramamine	antihistamine
dimethothiazine	Banistyl	antihistamine
dinoprostone	Prostin E$_2$	uterine stimulant
diphenhydramine	Benadryl	antihistamine
diphenoxylate	Lomotil	diarrhoea
diphenylpyraline	Histryl	antihistamine
diprophylline	Silbephylline	bronchodilator
dipyridamole	Persantin	vasodilator
disodium etidronate	Didronel	Paget's disease
disopyramide	Rythmodan; Norpace	anti-arrhythmic
distigmine	Ubretid	anticholinesterase
disulfiram	Antabuse	alcoholism
dobutamine	Dobutrex	cardiac stimulant
domperidone	Motilium	anti-emetic
dopamine	Intropin	cardiac stimulant
dothiepin	Prothiaden	antidepressant
doxapram	Dopram	respiratory stimulant
doxepin	Sinequan	antidepressant
doxorubicin	Adriamycin	antibiotic
doxycycline	Vibramycin	antibiotic
droperidol	Droleptan	neuroleptic
drostanolone	Masteril	antineoplastic

Approved Name	Proprietary Name	Main Action, Type of Drug or Use
dydrogesterone	Duphaston	progestogen
econazole	Ecostatin	antifungal agent
ecothiopate	Phospholine	glaucoma
edrophonium	Tensilon	anticholinesterase
emepronium	Cetiprin	anticholinergic
ergotamine	Lingraine	migraine
erythromycin	Erythrocin; Ilotycin	antibiotic
estramustine	Estracyt	antineoplastic
etamiphylline	Millophyline	bronchodilator
ethacrynic acid	Edecrin	diuretic
ethambutol	Myambutol	tuberculosis
ethamivan	Clairvan	respiratory stimulant
ethamsylate	Dicynene	haemostatic
ethionamide	Trescatyl	tuberculosis
ethoglucid	Epodyl	antineoplastic
ethosuximide	Emeside; Zarontin	anticonvulsant
ethotoin	Peganone	anticonvulsant
ethyloestrenol	Orabolin	anabolic steroid
etomidate	Hypnomidate	i.v. anaesthetic
etoposide	Vepesid	antineoplastic
etretinate	Tigason	psoriasis
fazadinium	Fazadon	muscle relaxant
fenbufen	Lederfen	antirheumatic
fenclofenac	Flenac	antirheumatic
fenfluramine	Ponderax	appetite depressant

144

fenoprofen	Fenopron; Progesic	antirheumatic
fenoterol	Berotec	bronchodilator
fentanyl	Sublimaze	analgesic
feprazone	Methrazone	antirheumatic
flavoxate	Urispas	antispasmodic
fluclorolone	Topilar	corticosteroid
flucloxacillin	Floxapen	antibiotic
fludrocortisone	Florinef	corticosteroid
flufenamic acid	Meralen	antirheumatic
flumethasone	Locorten	corticosteroid
flunisolide	Syntaris	rhinitis
fluocinolone	Synalar	corticosteroid
fluocinonide	Metosyn	corticosteroid
fluocortolone	Ultralanum	corticosteroid
flupenthixol	Depixol; Fluanoxol	schizophrenia; antidepressant
fluphenazine	Moditen; Modecate	tranquilliser
flurandrenolone	Haelan	corticosteroid
flurazepam	Dalmane	soporific
flurbiprofen	Froben	antirheumatic
fluspirilene	Redeptin	tranquilliser
fosfestrol	Honvan	antineoplastic
framycetin	Framygen; Soframycin	antibiotic
frusemide	Dryptal; Lasix	diuretic
furazolidone	Furoxone	intestinal antiseptic
gallamine	Flaxedil	muscle relaxant
gentamicin	Cidomycin; Genticin; Alcomicin	antibiotic

145

Approved Name	Proprietary Name	Main Action, Type of Drug or Use
gestronol	Depostat	prostatic hyperplasia
glibenclamide	Daonil; Euglucon	oral hypoglycaemic
glibornuride	Glutril	oral hypoglycaemic
gliclazide	Diamicron	oral hypoglycaemic
glipizide	Glibenese, Minodiab	oral hypoglycaemic
gliquidone	Glurenorm	oral hypoglycaemic
glutaraldehyde	Glutarol	warts
glutethimide	Doriden	hypnotic
glymidine	Gondafon	oral hypoglycaemic
griseofulvin	Fulcin; Grisovin	antifungal antibiotic
guanethidine	Ismelin	antihypertensive
guanoclor	Vatensol	antihypertensive
halcinonide	Halciderm	corticosteroid
haloperidol	Haldol; Serenace	tranquilliser
halothane	Fluothane	anaesthetic
heparin	Pularin	anticoagulant
heptabarbitone	Medomin	hypnotic
hexamine hippurate	Hiprex	urinary antiseptic
hexamine mandelate	Mandelamine	urinary antiseptic
hyaluronidase	Hyalase	enzyme
hydralazine	Apresoline	antihypertensive
hydrargaphen	Penotrane	antiseptic
hydrochlorothiazide	Direma; Esidrex; Hydrosaluric	diuretic
hydrocortisone	Ef-Cortelan; Hydro-cortistab; Hydrocortone	corticosteroid

hydroflumethiazide	Hydrenox	diuretic
hydroxocobalamin	Neo-Cytamen	anti-anaemic
hydroxychloroquine	Plaquenil	antimalarial
hydroxyprogesterone	Proluton-Depot	progestogen
hydroxyurea	Hydrea	antineoplastic
hydroxyzine	Atarax	tranquilliser
ibuprofen	Brufen	antirheumatic
idoxuridine	Kerecid; Dendrid; Herpid	antiviral
ifosfamide	Mitoxana	antineoplastic
imipramine	Tofranil	antidepressant
indapamide	Natrilix	hypertension
indomethacin	Indocid; Imbrilon	antirheumatic
indoramin	Baratol	hypertension
inositol nicotinate	Hexopal	vasodilator
iodapamide	Biligrafin	contrast agent
iopanoic acid	Telepaque	contrast agent
iophendylate	Myodil	contrast agent
ipratropium	Atrovent	bronchodilator
iprindole	Prondol	antidepressant
iproniazid	Marsilid	antidepressant
isoaminile	Dimyril	antitussive
isocarboxazid	Marplan	antidepressant
isoetharine	Numotac	bronchodilator
isoprenaline	Aleudrin; Saventrine	bronchodilator
isosorbide dinitrate	Cedocard; Vascardin	angina
isoxsuprine	Duvadilan; Defencin	vasodilator
kanamycin	Kannasyn; Kantrex	antibiotic

147

Approved Name	Proprietary Name	Main Action, Type of Drug or Use
ketamine	Ketalar	anaesthetic
ketazolam	Anxon	tranquilliser
ketoconazole	Nizoral	antifungal
ketoprofen	Orudis	antirheumatic
ketotifen	Zaditen	anti-asthmatic
labetalol	Trandate	hypertension
lactulose	Duphalac; Gatinar	laxative
lanatoside C	Cedilanid	cardiac stimulant
levallorphan	Lorfan	narcotic antagonist
levodopa	Brocadopa; Larodopa	parkinsonism
levorphanol	Dromoran	analgesic
lidoflazine	Clinium	angina
lignocaine	Xylocaine; Xylocard; Xylotox	anaesthetic
lincomycin	Lincocin	antibiotic
liothyronine	Tertroxin	thyroid hormone
lomustine	CCNU	antineoplastic
loperamide	Imodium	antidiarrhoeal
lorazepam	Ativan	antidepressant
lormetazepam	Noctamid	soporific
lymecycline	Tetralysal	antibiotic
malathion	Derbac; Prioderm	parasiticide
maprotiline	Ludiomil	antidepressant
mazindol	Teronac	appetite depressant
mebendazole	Vermox	anthelmintic

mebeverine	Colofac	antispasmodic
mebhydrolin	Fabahistin	antihistamine
mecamylamine	Inversine	antihypertensive
mecillinam	Selexidin	antibiotic
medazepam	Nobrium	tranquilliser
medigoxin	Lanitop	cardiac stimulant
medroxyprogesterone	Provera	progestogen
mefenamic acid	Ponstan	antirheumatic
mefruside	Baycaron	diuretic
melphalan	Alkeran	antineoplastic
menadiol	Synkavit	hypoprothrombinaemia
menotrophin	Perganol	hypogonadism
mepenzolate	Cantil	intestinal sedative
mepivacaine	Chlorocain	anaesthetic
meprobamate	Equanil; Miltown	tranquilliser
mepyramine	Anthisan	antihistamine
mequitazine	Primalan	antihistamine
mercaptopurine	Puri-Nethol	antineoplastic
mesterolone	Pro-Viron	androgen
metaraminol	Aramine	hypertensive
metformin	Glucophage	oral hypoglycaemic
methacycline	Rondomycin	antibiotic
methadone	Physeptone	analgesic
methicillin	Celbenin	antibiotic
methixene	Tremonil	parkinsonism
methocarbamol	Robaxin	muscle relaxant
methohexitone	Brietal	anaesthetic

Approved Name	Proprietary Name	Main Action, Type of Drug or Use
methoserpidine	Decaserpyl	antihypertensive
methotrexate	Emtexate	antineoplastic
methoxamine	Vasoxine	vasoconstrictor
methoxyflurane	Penthrane	anaesthetic
methoxyphenamine	Orthoxine	bronchodilator
methyclothiazide	Enduron	diuretic
methylcysteine	Visclair	mucolytic
methyldopa	Aldomet	antihypertensive
methylphenidate	Ritalin	stimulant
methylphenobarbitone	Prominal	epilepsy
methylprednisolone	Medrone	corticosteroid
methyprylone	Noludar	hypnotic
methysergide	Deseril	vasoconstrictor
metoclopramide	Maxolon; Primperan	anti-emetic
metolazone	Metenix	hypertension
metoprolol	Betaloc; Lopresor	adrenergic blockade
metronidazole	Flagyl	trichomoniasis
metyrapone	Metopirone	enzyme inhibitor
mexenone	Uvistat	sunscreen
mexiletine	Mexitil	cardiac arrhythmia
mezlocillin	Baypen	antibiotic
mianserin	Bolvidon; Norval	antidepressant
miconazole	Daktarin	antifungal
minocycline	Minocin	antibiotic
minoxidil	Loniten	hypertension

mitobronitol	Myelobromol	antineoplastic
nadolol	Corgard	hypertension
naftidrofuryl	Praxilene	vasodilator
nalidixic acid	Negram	urinary antiseptic
naloxone	Narcan	narcotic antagonist
nandrolone	Deca-Durabolin; Durabolin	anabolic steroid
naproxen	Naprosyn	antirheumatic
natamycin	Pimafucin	antibiotic
nefopam	Acupan	analgesic
neostigmine	Prostigmin	myasthenia gravis
netilmicin	Netillin	antibiotic
niclosamide	Yomesan	anthelmintic
nicofuranose	Bradilan	vasodilator
nicotinyl alcohol	Ronicol	vasodilator
nicoumalone	Sinthrome	anticoagulant
nifedipine	Adalat	angina
nimorazole	Naxogin	trichomoniasis
niridazole	Ambilhar	schistosomiasis
nitrazepam	Mogadon	soporific
nitrofurantoin	Furadantin	urinary antiseptic
nitrofurazone	Furacin	antiseptic
nomifensine	Merital	antidepressant
noradrenaline	Levophed	hypertensive
norethandrolone	Nilevar	anabolic steroid
norethisterone	Primolut N	progestogen
nortriptyline	Allegron; Aventyl	antidepressant
novobiocin	Albamycin T	antibiotic

Approved Name	Proprietary Name	Main Action, Type of Drug or Use
noxythiolin	Noxyflex S	antiseptic
nystatin	Nystan	antifungal antibiotic
orciprenaline	Alupent	bronchodilator
orphenadrine	Disipal	parkinsonism
oxazepam	Serenid	tranquilliser
oxedrine	Sympatol	vasoconstrictor
oxpentifylline	Trental	vasodilator
oxprenolol	Trasicor	adrenergic blockade
oxymetazoline	Afrazine	nasal decongestant
oxymetholone	Anapolon	anabolic steroid
oxypertine	Integrin	tranquilliser
oxyphenbutazone	Tanderil	antirheumatic
oxytetracycline	Berkmycen; Imperacin; Terramycin	antibiotic
oxytocin	Pitocin; Syntocinon	induction of labour
pancuronium	Pavulon	muscle relaxant
paracetamol	Calpol; Panadol	analgesic
paramethadione	Paradione	anticonvulsant
pargyline	Eutonyl	antihypertensive
pemoline	Volital; Ronyl	cerebral stimulant
penicillamine	Distamine; Cuprimine	chelating agent
pentaerythritol tetranitrate	Mycardol; Peritrate	coronary dilator
pentagastrin	Peptavlon	gastric stimulant
pentazocine	Fortral	analgesic
penthienate	Monodral	antispasmodic

152

perhexiline	Pexid	angina
pericyazine	Neulactil	tranquilliser
perphenazine	Fentazin	tranquilliser
phenazocine	Narphen	analgesic
phenazopyridine	Pyridium	urinary analgesic
phenelzine	Nardil	antidepressant
phenethicillin	Broxil	antibiotic
phenformin	Dibotin	oral hypoglycaemic
phenindamine	Thephorin	antihistamine
phenindione	Dindevan	anticoagulant
pheniramine	Daneral	antihistamine
phenoperidine	Operidine	analgesic
phenoxybenzamine	Dibenyline	adrenaline antagonist
phenoxymethylpenicillin	Crystapen V; Distaquaine V-K; V-Cil-K	antibiotic
phentermine	Duromine; Ionamin	appetite depressant
phentolamine	Rogitine	adrenaline antagonist
phenylbutazone	Butazolidin	antirheumatic
phenylephrine	Neophryn	decongestant
phenytoin	Epanutin	epilepsy
phthalylsulphathiazole	Thalazole	sulphonamide
phytomenadione	Konakion	hypoprothrombinaemia
pimozide	Orap	tranquilliser
pindolol	Visken	coronary dilator
pipenzolate	Piptal	antispasmodic
piperacillin	Pipril	antibiotic
piperazine	Antepar	anthelmintic

Approved Name	Proprietary Name	Main Action, Type of Drug or Use
piritramide	Dipidolor	analgesic
piroxicam	Feldene	antirheumatic
pivampicillin	Pondocillin	antibiotic
pivmecillinam	Selexid	antibiotic
pizotifen	Sanomigran	migraine
poldine	Nacton	antispasmodic
polymyxin B	Aerosporin	antibiotic
polynoxylin	Anaflex	antiseptic
polythiazide	Nephril	diuretic
prazepam	Centrax	tranquilliser
prazosin	Hypovase	antihypertensive
prednisolone	Codelcortone; Deltacortril; Deltastab; PreCortisyl; Prednesol	corticosteroid
prednisone	DeCortisyl; Deltacortone	corticosteroid
prenalterol	Hyprenan; Varbian	B$_1$-adrenoceptor stimulant
prenylamine	Synadrin	coronary dilator
prilocaine	Citanest	anaesthetic
primidone	Mysoline	anticonvulsant
probenecid	Benemid	uricosuric
probucol	Lurselle	hypercholesterolaemia
procainamide	Pronestyl	myocardial depressant
procaine-penicillin	Depocillin	antibiotic
procarbazine	Natulan	antineoplastic
prochlorperazine	Stemetil	tranquilliser

154

procyclidine	Kemadrin	parkinsonism
proguanil	Paludrine	antimalarial
promazine	Sparine	tranquilliser
promethazine	Phenergan	antihistamine
promethazine theoclate	Avomine	anti-emetic
propanidid	Epontol	anaesthetic
propantheline bromide	Pro-Banthine	anticholinergic
propranolol	Inderal	adrenergic blockade
propyliodone	Dionosil	contrast agent
prothionamide	Trevintix	tuberculosis
protriptyline	Concordin	antidepressant
pyrazinamide	Zinamide	tuberculosis
pyridostigmine	Mestinon	myasthenia gravis
pyrimethamine	Daraprim	antimalarial
quinalbarbitone sodium	Seconal Sodium	hypnotic
quinestradol	Pentovis	oestrogen
quinethazone	Aquamox	diuretic
ranitidine	Zantac	peptic ulcer
razoxane	Razoxane	antineoplastic
reserpine	Serpasil	antihypertensive
rifampicin	Rifadin; Rimactane	antibiotic
rimiterol	Pulmadil	bronchodilator
ritodrine	Yutopar	premature labour
salbutamol	Ventolin	bronchodilator
salcatonin	Calsynar	Paget's disease
salsalate	Disalcid	antirheumatic
silver sulphadiazine	Flamazine	antibacterial

Approved Name	Proprietary Name	Main Action, Type of Drug or Use
sodium acetrizoate	Diaginol	contrast agent
sodium cromoglycate	Intal; Rynacrom; Nalcrom	anti-allergic
sodium diatrizoate	Hypaque	contrast agent
sodium fusidate	Fucidin	antibiotic
sodium ipodate	Biloptin	contrast agent
sodium ironedetate	Sytron	anti-anaemic
sodium nitroprusside	Nipride	hypertensive crisis
sodium picosulphate	Laxoberal	laxative
sodium valproate	Epilim	epilepsy
sotalol	Beta-Cardone; Sotacor	adrenergic blockade
spectinomycin	Trobicin	antibiotic
spironolactone	Aldactone; Spiroctan	diuretic
stanozolol	Stromba	anabolic steroid
sulfadoxine	Fanosil	antimalarial
sulfametopyrazine	Kelfizine	sulphonamide
sulindac	Clinoril	arthritis
sulphacetamide	Albucid	sulphonamide
sulphadimethoxine	Madribon	sulphonamide
sulphadimidine	Sulphamezathine	sulphonamide
sulphafurazole	Gantrisin	sulphonamide
sulphamethizole	Urolucosil	sulphonamide
sulphamethoxypyridazine	Lederkyn	sulphonamide
sulphaphenazole	Orisulf	sulphonamide
sulphasalazine	Salazopyrin	sulphonamide
sulphathiazole	Thiazamide	sulphonamide

sulphinpyrazone	Anturan	uricosuric
sulthiame	Ospolot	anticonvulsant
suxamethonium bromide	Brevidil M	muscle relaxant
suxamethonium chloride	Anectine; Scoline	muscle relaxant
talampicillin	Talpen	antibiotic
tamoxifen	Nolvadex	antineoplastic
temazepam	Euhypnos; Normison	soporific
terbutaline	Bricanyl	bronchodilator
terfenadine	Triludan	antihistamine
tetracosactrin	Synacthen	corticotrophin
tetracycline	Achromycin; Tetrachel; Tetracyn	antibiotic
thiabendazole	Mintezol	anthelmintic
thiambutosine	Ciba 1906	antileprotic
thiethylperazine	Torecan	anti-emetic
thioguanine	Lanvis	antineoplastic
thiomersal	Merthiolate	antiseptic
thiopentone	Intraval	i.v. anaesthetic
thiopropazate	Dartalan	tranquilliser
thioridazine	Melleril	tranquilliser
thymoxamine	Opilon	vasodilator
thyroxine	Eltroxin	thyroid deficiency
ticarcillin	Ticar	antibiotic
tigloidine	Tiglyssin	spasticity
timolol	Blocadren; Betim	adrenergic blockade
tobramycin	Nebcin	antibiotic
tocainide	Tonocard	anti-arrhythmic

Approved Name	Proprietary Name	Main Action, Type of Drug or Use
tofenacin	Elamol	antidepressant
tolazamide	Tolanase	oral hypoglycaemic
tolazoline	Priscol	vasodilator
tolbutamide	Rastinon	oral hypoglycaemic
tolmetin	Tolectin	antirheumatic
tolnaftate	Tinaderm	antimycotic
tranexamic acid	Cyklokapron	antifibrinolytic
tranylcypromine	Parnate	antidepressant
trazodone	Molipaxin	antidepressant
tretinoin	Retin-A	acne
triamcinolone	Adcortyl; Ledercort	corticosteroid
triamterene	Dytac	diuretic
triazolam	Halcion	soporific
trifluoperazine	Stelazine	tranquilliser
trilostane	Modrenal	aldosteronism
trimeprazine	Vallergan	antihistamine
trimetaphan	Arfonad	antihypertensive
trimethoprim	Syraprim; Trimopan	antibacterial
trimipramine	Surmontil	antidepressant
triprolidine	Actidil	antihistamine
tropicamide	Mydriacyl	mydriatic
tryptophan	Pacitron	antidepressant
troxidone	Tridione	anticonvulsant
tubocurarine	Tubarine	muscle relaxant
tyloxapol	Alevaire	mucolytic

urokinase	Ukidan; Abbokinase	thrombolytic
ursodeoxycholic acid	Destolit	gallstones
vancomycin	Vancocin	antibiotic
verapamil	Cordilox	angina
vidarabine	Vira-A	antineoplastic
viloxazine	Vivalan	antidepressant
vinblastine	Velbe	antineoplastic
vincristine	Oncovin	antineoplastic
vindesine	Eldisine	antineoplastic
warfarin	Marevan	anticoagulant
xipamide	Diurexan	diuretic
xylometazoline	Otrivine	decongestant
zimelidine	Zelmid	antidepressant
zomepirac	Zomax	analgesic

159

Proprietary Name	Approved Name	Main Action, Type of Drug or Use
Abbokinase	urokinase	thrombolytic
Achromycin	tetracycline	antibiotic
Acthar	corticotrophin	hormone
Actidil	triprolidine	antihistamine
Acupan	nefopam	analgesic
Adalat	nifedipine	angina
Adcortyl	triamcinolone	corticosteroid
Adriamycin	doxorubicin	antibiotic
Aerosporin	polymyxin B	antibiotic
Afrazine	oxymetazoline	nasal decongestant
Airbron	acetylcysteine	mucolytic
Akineton	biperiden	parkinsonism
Albamycin T	novobiocin	antibiotic
Albucid	sulphacetamide	sulphonamide
Alcomicin	gentamicin	antibiotic
Alcopar	bephenium	anthelmintic
Aldactone	spironolactone	diuretic
Aldomet	methyldopa	antihypertensive
Aleudrin	isoprenaline	bronchodilator
Alevaire	tyloxapol	mucolytic
Alkeran	melphalan	antineoplastic
Allegron	nortriptyline	antidepressant
Alloferin	alcuronium	muscle relaxant
Alupent	orciprenaline	bronchodilator
Ambaxin	bacampicillin	antibiotic

Ambilhar	niridazole	anthelmintic
Amfipen	ampicillin	antibiotic
Amikin	amikacin	antibiotic
Amoxil	amoxycillin	antibiotic
Amytal	amylobarbitone	hypnotic
Anaflex	polynoxylin	antiseptic
Anafranil	clomipramine	antidepressant
Anapolon	oxymetholone	anabolic steroid
Androcur	cyproterone	pituitary suppressant
Anectine	suxamethonium	muscle relaxant
Anquil	benperidol	tranquilliser
Antabuse	disulfiram	alcoholism
Antepar	piperazine	anthelmintic
Anthisan	mepyramine	antihistamine
Anturan	sulphinpyrazone	uricosuric
Anxon	ketazolam	tranquilliser
Apresoline	hydralazine	antihypertensive
Aprinox	bendrofluazide	diuretic
Aquamox	quinethazone	diuretic
Aramine	metaraminol	hypotensive
Arfonad	trimetaphan	antihypertensive
Artane	benzhexol	parkinsonism
Arvin	ancrod	anticoagulant
AT10	dihydrotachysterol	hypocalcaemia
Atarax	hydroxyzine	tranquilliser
Atensine	diazepam	tranquilliser; muscle relaxant
Ativan	lorazepam	antidepressant

Proprietary Name	Approved Name	Main Action, Type of Drug or Use
Atromid-S	clofibrate	hypercholesterolaemia
Atrovent	ipratropium	antibiotic
Aureomycin	chlortetracycline	antibiotic
Aventyl	nortriptyline	antidepressant
Avloclor	chloroquine	antimalarial
Avomine	promethazine theoclate	anti-emetic
Banistyl	dimethothiazine	antihistamine
Banocide	diethylcarbamazine	filaricide
Baratol	indoramin	hypertension
Baycaron	mefruside	diuretic
Baypen	mezlocillin	antibiotic
Becotide	beclomethasone	corticosteroid
Benadryl	diphenhydramine	antihistamine
Benemid	probenecid	uricosuric
Benoral	benorylate	analgesic
Berkmycen	oxytetracycline	antibiotic
Berotec	fenoterol	bronchodilator
Beta-Cardone	sotalol	adrenergic blockade
Betaloc	metoprolol	adrenergic blockade
Betim	timolol	adrenergic blockade
Betnelan	betamethasone	corticosteroid
BICNU	carmustine	antineoplastic
Biligrafin	iodipamide	contrast agent
Biloptin	sodium ipodate	contrast agent
Biogastrone	carbenoxolone	peptic ulcer

Bisolvon	bromhexine	mucolytic
Blocadren	timolol	adrenergic blockade
Bolvidon	mianserin	antidepressant
Bradilan	nicofuranose	vasodilator
Bretylate	bretylium	arrhythmias
Brevidil	suxamethonium	muscle relaxant
Bricanyl	terbutaline	bronchodilator
Brietal	methohexitone	anaesthetic
Brinaldix	clopamide	diuretic
Brocadopa	levodopa	parkinsonism
Broxil	phenethicillin	antibiotic
Brufen	ibuprofen	antirheumatic
Burinex	bumetanide	diuretic
Butazolidin	phenylbutazone	antirheumatic
CCNU	lomustine	antineoplastic
Calcitare	calcitonin	hormone
Calciparine	calcium heparin	anticoagulant
Calpol	paracetamol	analgesic
Calsynar	salcatonin	**Paget's disease**
Calthor	ciclacillin	antibiotic
Camcolit	lithium carbonate	mania
Candeptin	candicidin	antibiotic
Canestan	clotrimazole	antimycotic
Cantil	mepenzolate	intestinal sedative
Capastat	capreomycin	tuberculosis
Caplenal	allopurinol	uricosuric
Capoten	captopril	severe hypertension

Proprietary Name	Approved Name	Main Action, Type of Drug or Use
Carisoma	carisoprodol	muscle relaxant
Carylderm	carbaryl	parasiticide
Catapres	clonidine	hypertension
Cedelanid	lanatoside C	cardiac stimulant
Cedocard	isosorbide dinitrate	angina
Celbenin	methicillin	antibiotic
Centrax	prazepam	antidepressant
Centyl	bendrofluazide	diuretic
Ceporex	cephalexin	antibiotic
Ceporin	cephaloridine	antibiotic
Cetiprin	emepronium	anticholinergic
Chendol	chenodeoxycholic acid	gallstone solvent
Chloromycetin	chloramphenicol	antibiotic
Choledyl	choline theophyllinate	bronchodilator
Ciba 1906	thiambutosine	antileprotic
Cidomycin	gentamicin	antibiotic
Cinobac	cinoxacin	antibiotic
Citanest	prilocaine	anaesthetic
Claforan	cefotaxime	antibiotic
Clairvan	ethamivan	respiratory stimulant
Clinium	lidoflazine	angina
Clinoril	sulindac	rheumatoid disease
Clomid	clomiphene	infertility
Clopixol	clopenthixol	schizophrenia
Codelcortone	prednisolone	corticosteroid

Cogentin	benztropine	parkinsonism
Colestid	colestipol	exchange resin
Colofac	mebeverine	antispasmodic
Colomycin	colistin	antibiotic
Concordin	protriptyline	antidepressant
Cordilox	verapamil	angina
Corgard	nadolol	hypertension
Cortef	hydrocortisone	corticosteroid
Cortelan	cortisone	corticosteroid
Cortril	hydrocortisone	corticosteroid
Cosmegen	actinomycin D	antineoplastic
Crystapen V	phenoxymethylpenicillin	antibiotic
Cuprimine	penicillamine	chelating agent
Cyclospasmol	cyclandelate	vasodilator
Cyklokapron	tranexamic acid	antifibrinolytic
Cytacon	cyanocobalamin	anti-anaemic
Cytamen	cyanocobalamin	anti-anaemic
Cytosar	cytarabine	antineoplastic
DDAVP	desmopressin	diabetes insipidus
DF 118	dihydrocodeine	analgesic
DTIC	dacarbazine	antineoplastic
Daktarin	miconazole	antifungal
Dalacin C	clindamycin	antibiotic
Dalmane	flurazepam	soporific
Daneral	pheniramine	antihistamine
Danol	danazol	pituitary depressant
Dantrium	dantrolene	muscle relaxant

Proprietary Name	Approved Name	Main Action, Type of Drug or Use
Daonil	glibenclamide	oral hypoglycaemic
Daranide	dichlorphenamide	glaucoma
Daraprim	pyrimethamine	antimalarial
Dartalan	thiopropazate	tranquilliser
Decadron	dexamethasone	corticosteroid
Deca-Durabolin	nandrolone	anabolic steroid
Decaserpyl	methoserpidine	antihypertensive
Declinax	debrisoquine	antihypertensive
Decortisyl	prednisone	corticosteroid
Defencin	isoxuprine	vasodilator
Deltacortone	prednisone	corticosteroid
Deltacortril	prednisolone	corticosteroid
Dendrid	idoxuridine	antiviral
Depixol	flupenthixol	schizophrenia
Depocillin	procaine-penicillin	antibiotic
Depostat	gestronol	prostatic hyperplasia
Derbac	carbaryl	parasiticide
Dermovate	clobetasol	corticosteroid
Deseril	methysergide	vasoconstrictor
Desferal	desferrioxamine	chelating agent
Destolit	ursodeoxycholic acid	gallstones
Dexacortisyl	dexamethasone	corticosteroid
Dexedrine	dexamphetamine	appetite depressant
Dextraven	dextran	plasma substitute
Diabinese	chlorpropamide	oral hypoglycaemic

Diaginol	sodium acetrizoate — contrast agent
Diamicron	gliclazide — oral hypoglycaemic
Diamox	acetazolamide — glaucoma
Dibenyline	phenoxybenzamine — adrenaline antagonist
Dibotin	phenformin — oral hypoglycaemic
Dicynene	ethamsylate — haemostatic
Didronel	disodium etidronate — Paget's disease
Dihydergot	dihydroergotamine — migraine
Dimelor	acetohexamide — oral hypoglycaemic
Dimotane	brompheniramine — antihistamine
Dindevan	phenindione — anticoagulant
Dionosil	propyliodone — contrast agent
Dipidolor	piritramide — analgesic
Direma	hydrochlorothiazide — diuretic
Disalcid	salsalate — antirheumatic
Disipal	orphenadrine — parkinsonism
Distaclor	cefaclor — antibiotic
Distamine	penicillamine — chelating agent
Distaquaine V-K	phenoxymethylpenicillin — antibiotic
Diurexan	xipamide — diuretic
Dixarit	clonidine — antihypertensive; migraine
Dobutrex	dobutamine — cardiac stimulant
Dolobid	diflunisal — analgesic
Doloxene	dextropropoxyphene — analgesic
Dopram	doxapram — respiratory stimulant
Dorbanex	danthron — laxative
Doriden	glutethimide — hypnotic

Proprietary Name	Approved Name	Main Action, Type of Drug or Use
Dramamine	dimenhydrinate	antihistamine
Droleptan	droperidol	analgesic
Dromoran	levorphanol	analgesic
Dryptal	frusemide	diuretic
Dulcolax	bisacodyl	laxative
Duogastrone	carbenoxolone	peptic ulcer
Duphalac	lactulose	laxative
Duphaston	dydrogesterone	progestogen
Durabolin	nandrolone	anabolic steroid
Duromine	phentermine	appetite depressant
Duvadilan	isoxsuprine	vasodilator
Dytac	triamterene	diuretic
Ecostatin	econazole	antifungal agent
Edecrin	ethacrynic acid	diuretic
Ef-cortelan	hydrocortisone	corticosteroid
Elamol	tofenacin	antidepressant
Eldesine	vindesine	antineoplastic
Eltroxin	thyroxine	thyroid deficiency
Emeside	ethosuximide	anticonvulsant
Emtexate	methotrexate	antineoplastic
Endoxana	cyclophosphamide	antineoplastic
Enduron	methyclothiazide	diuretic
Epanutin	phenytoin	epilepsy
Epilim	sodium valproate	epilepsy
Epodyl	ethoglucid	antineoplastic

Epontol	propanidid	anaesthetic
Epsikapron	aminocaproic acid	haemostatic
Equanil	meprobamate	tranquilliser
Eradicin	acrosoxacin, rosoxacin	gonorrhoea
Erythrocin	erythromycin	antibiotic
Esbatal	bethanidine	antihypertensive
Esidrex	hydrochlorothiazide	diuretic
Estracyt	estramustine	antineoplastic
Etophylate	acepifylline	bronchodilator
Eudemine	diazoxide	antihypertensive
Euglucon	glibenclamide	oral hypoglycaemic
Euhypnos	temazepam	soporific
Eumovate	clobetasone	corticosteroid
Eurax	crotamiton	antipruritic
Eutonyl	pargyline	antihypertensive
Evadyne	butriptyline	antidepressant
Fabahistin	mebhydrolin	antihistamine
Fanosil	sulphadoxine	antimalarial
Fazadon	fazadinium	muscle relaxant
Feldene	piroxicam	antirheumatic
Fenopron	fenoprofen	antirheumatic
Fentazin	perphenazine	tranquilliser
Flagyl	metronidazole	trichomoniasis
Flamazine	silver sulphadiazine	antibacterial
Flaxedil	gallamine	muscle relaxant
Flenac	fenclofenac	antirheumatic
Florinef	fludrocortisone	corticosteroid

Proprietary Name	Approved Name	Main Action, Type of Drug or Use
Floxapen	flucloxacillin	antibiotic
Fluanoxol	flupenthixol	antidepressant
Fluothane	halothane	anaesthetic
Fortral	pentazocine	analgesic
Framygen	framycetin	antibiotic
Frisium	clobazam	tranquilliser
Froben	flurbiprofen	rheumatoid disease
Fucidin	sodium fusidate	antibiotic
Fulcin	griseofulvin	antifungal antibiotic
Fungilin	amphotericin	antifungal antibiotic
Fungizone	amphotericin	antifungal antibiotic
Furacin	nitrofurazone	antiseptic
Furadantin	nitrofurantoin	urinary antiseptic
Furoxone	furazolidone	intestinal antiseptic
Gantrisin	sulphafurazole	sulphonamide
Gatinar	lactulose	laxative
Genticin	gentamicin	antibiotic
Gestanin	allyloestrenol	progestogen
Glibenese	glipizide	oral hypoglycaemic
Glucophage	metformin	oral hypoglycaemic
Glurenorm	gliquidone	oral hypoglycaemic
Glutril	glibornuride	oral hypoglycaemic
Gondafon	glymidine	oral hypoglycaemic
Grisovin	griseofulvin	antifungal antibiotic
Haelan	flurandrenolone	corticosteroid

Halciderm	halcinonide	corticosteroid
Halcion	triazolam	soporific
Haldol	haloperidol	schizophrenia
Harmonyl	deserpidine	antihypertensive
Heminevrin	chlormethiazole	soporific
Herpid	idoxuridine	antiviral
Hexopal	inositol nicotinate	vasodilator
Hibitane	chlorhexidine	antiseptic
Hiprex	hexamine hippurate	urinary antiseptic
Histryl	diphenylpyraline	antihistamine
Honvan	fosfestrol	antineoplastic
Hyalase	hyaluronidase	enzyme
Hydrea	hydroxyurea	antineoplastic
Hydrenox	hydroflumethiazide	diuretic
Hydrocortisyl	hydrocortisone	corticosteroid
Hydrocortone	hydrocortisone	corticosteroid
HydroSaluric	hydrochlorothiazide	diuretic
Hygroton	chlorthalidone	diuretic
Hypaque	sodium diatrizoate	contrast agent
Hypnomidate	etomidate	i.v. anaesthetic
Hypovase	prazosin	antihypertensive
Hyprenan	prenalterol	B_1-adrenoceptor stimulant
Icipen	phenoxymethylpenicillin	antibiotic
Ilosone	erythromycin estolate	antibiotic
Ilotycin	erythromycin	antibiotic
Imbrilon	indomethacin	antirheumatic
Imodium	loperamide	antidiarrhoeal

Proprietary Name	Approved Name	Main Action, Type of Drug or Use
Imperacin	oxytetracycline	antibiotic
Imuran	azathioprine	immunosuppressive
Inderal	propranolol	adrenergic blockade
Indocid	indomethacin	antirheumatic
Intal	sodium cromoglycate	anti-asthmatic
Integrin	oxypertine	tranquilliser
Intraval	thiopentone	i.v. anaesthetic
Intropin	dopamine	cardiac stimulant
Inversine	mecamylamine	antihypertensive
Ionamin	phenteramine	appetite depressant
Ismelin	guanethidine	antihypertensive
Isordil	isosorbide dinitrate	angina
Kannasyn	kanamycin	antibiotic
Kantrex	kanamycin	antibiotic
Kefadol	cefamandole	antibiotic
Keflex	cephalexin	antibiotic
Keflin	cephalothin	antibiotic
Kefzol	cephazolin	antibiotic
Kelfizine	sulfametopyrazine	sulphonamide
Kelocyanor	dicobalt edetate	cyanide poisoning
Kemadrin	procyclidine	parkinsonism
Kerecid	idoxuridine	antiviral
Konakion	phytomenadione	hypoprothrombinaemia
Lamprene	clofazimine	antileprotic
Lanitop	medigoxin	cardiac stimulant

172

Lanoxin	digoxin	cardiac failure
Lanvis	thioguanine	antineoplastic
Largactil	chlorpromazine	tranquilliser
Larodopa	levodopa	parkinsonism
Lasix	frusemide	diuretic
Laxoberal	sodium picosulphate	laxative
Ledercort	triamcinolone	corticosteroid
Lederfen	fenbufen	antirheumatic
Lederkyn	sulphamethoxypyridazine	sulphonamide
Ledermycin	demeclocycline	antibiotic
Lentizol	amitriptyline	antidepressant
Leukeran	chlorambucil	antineoplastic
Levophed	noradrenaline	hypertensive
Librium	chlordiazepoxide	tranquilliser
Lincocin	lincomycin	antibiotic
Lioresal	baclofen	muscle relaxant
Locorten	flumethasone	corticosteroid
Loniten	minoxidil	hypertension
Lopresor	metoprolol	adrenergic blockade
Lorfan	levallorphan	narcotic antagonist
Ludiomil	maprotiline	antidepressant
Lurselle	probucol	hypercholesterolaemia
Lynoral	ethinyloestradiol	menopause
Madribon	sulphadimethoxine	sulphonamide
Mandelamine	hexamine mandelate	urinary antiseptic
Marcain	bupivacaine	anaesthetic
Marevan	warfarin	anticoagulant

Proprietary Name	Approved Name	Main Action, Type of Drug or Use
Marplan	isocarboxazid	antidepressant
Marsilid	iproniazid	antidepressant
Masteril	drostanolone	antineoplastic
Maxolon	metoclopramide	anti-emetic
Medomin	heptabarbitone	hypnotic
Medrone	methylprednisolone	corticosteroid
Mefoxin	cefoxitin	antibiotic
Megaclor	clomocycline	antibiotic
Megimide	bemigride	respiratory stimulant
Melitase	chlorpropamide	oral hypoglycaemic
Melleril	thioridazine	tranquilliser
Merbentyl	dicyclomine	antispasmodic
Merital	nomifensine	antidepressant
Merthiolate	thiomersal	antiseptic
Mestinon	pyridostigmine	myasthenia
Metenix	metolazone	hypertension
Methrazone	feprazone	antirheumatic
Metopirone	metyrapone	enzyme inhibitor
Metosyn	fluocinonide	corticosteroid
Mexitil	mexiletine	cardiac arrhythmias
Midamor	amiloride	diuretic
Millophyline	etamiphylline	bronchodilator
Miltown	meprobamate	tranquilliser
Minodiab	glipizide	oral hypoglycaemic
Minocin	minocycline	antibiotic

Mintezol	thiabendazole	anthelmintic
Mitoxana	ifosfamide	antineoplastic
Moditen	fluphenazine	tranquilliser
Modrenal	trilostane	aldosteronism
Mogadon	nitrazepam	soporific
Molipaxin	trazodone	antidepressant
Monodral	penthienate	antispasmodic
Motilium	domperidone	anti-emetic
Mucodyne	carbocisteine	mucolytic
Myambutol	ethambutol	tuberculosis
Mycardol	pentaerythritol tetranitrate	coronary dilator
Mydriacyl	tropicamide	mydriatic
Mydrilate	cyclopentolate	mydriatic
Myelobromol	mitobronitol	antineoplastic
Myleran	busulphan	antineoplastic
Myocrisin	sodium aurothiomalate	rheumatoid arthritis
Myodil	iophendylate	contrast agent
Mysoline	primidone	anticonvulsant
Mysteclin	tetracycline	antibiotic
Mytelase	ambenonium	myasthenia gravis
Nacton	poldine	antispasmodic
Nalcrom	sodium cromoglycate	ulcerative colitis
Naprosyn	naproxen	antirheumatic
Narcan	naloxone	narcotic antagonist
Nardil	phenelzine	antidepressant
Narphen	phenazocine	analgesic
Natrilix	indapamide	hypertension

Proprietary Name	Approved Name	Main Action, Type of Drug or Use
Natulan	procarbazine	antineoplastic
Navidrex	cyclopenthiazide	diuretic
Naxogin	nimorazole	trichomoniasis
Nebcin	tobramycin	antibiotic
Nefrolan	clorexolone	diuretic
Negram	nalidixic acid	urinary antiseptic
Neo-Cytamen	hydroxocobalamin	anti-anaemic
Neo-Mercazole	carbimazole	thyrotoxicosis
Neo-Naclex	bendrofluazide	diuretic
Neophryn	phenylephrine	decongestant
Neoplatin	cisplatin	antineoplastic
Nephril	polythiazide	diuretic
Nerisone	diflucortolone	corticosteroid
Netillin	netilmicin	antibiotic
Neulactil	pericyazine	tranquilliser
Nilevar	norethandrolone	anabolic steroid
Nipride	sodium nitroprusside	hypertensive crisis
Nivaquine	chloroquine	antimalarial
Nivemycin	neomycin	antibiotic
Nizoral	ketoconazole	antifungal
Nobrium	medazepam	tranquilliser
Noctamid	lormetazepam	soporific
Noludar	methyprylone	hypnotic
Nolvadex	tamoxifen	antineoplastic
Norflex	orphenadrine	muscle relaxant

Normison	temazepam	soporific
Norpace	disopyramide	cardiac arrythmias
Norval	mianserin	antidepressant
Noxyflex S	noxythiolin	antiseptic
Numotac	isoetharine	bronchodilator
Nupercaine	cinchocaine	anaesthetic
Nydrane	beclamide	anticonvulsant
Nystan	nystatin	antifungal antibiotic
Ocusol	sulphacetamide	sulphonamide
Oncovin	vincristine	antineoplastic
One-Alpha	alfacalcidol	vitamin D deficiency
Operidine	phenoperidine	analgesic
Opilon	thymoxamine	vasodilator
Opren	benoxaprofen	antirheumatic
Optimine	azatadine	antihistamine
Orabolin	ethylestrenol	anabolic steroid
Oradexon	dexamethasone	corticosteroid
Orap	pimozide	tranquilliser
Oratrol	dichlorphenamide	glaucoma
Orbenin	cloxacillin	antibiotic
Orisulf	sulphaphenazole	sulphonamide
Orthoxine	methoxyphenamine	bronchodilator
Orudis	ketoprofen	antirheumatic
Ospolot	sulthiame	anticonvulsant
Otrivine	xylometazoline	decongestant
Pacitron	tryptophan	antidepressant
Palfium	dextromoramide	analgesic

177

Proprietary Name	Approved Name	Main Action, Type of Drug or Use
Paludrine	proguanil	antimalarial
Panadol	paracetamol	analgesic
Paradione	paramethadione	anticonvulsant
Parlodel	bromocriptine	anti-lactation; acromegaly
Parnate	tranylcypromine	antidepressant
Parvolex	acetylcysteine	paracetamol overdose
Pavulon	pancuronium	muscle relaxant
Peganone	ethotoin	anticonvulsant
Penbritin	ampicillin	antibiotic
Penidural	benzathine penicillin	antibiotic
Penotrane	hydrargaphen	antiseptic
Penthrane	methoxyflurane	anaesthetic
Pentovis	quinestradol	oestrogen
Pentrexyl	ampicillin	antibiotic
Peptavlon	pentagastrin	gastric stimulant
Percorten M	deoxycortone	Addison's disease
Pergonal	menotrophin	hypogonadism
Periactin	cyproheptadine	antihistamine
Peritrate	pentaerythritol tetranitrate	coronary dilator
Peroidin	potassium perchlorate	hyperthyroidism
Persantin	dipyridamole	vasodilator
Pertofran	desipramine	antidepressant
Pexid	perhexiline	angina
Phanodorm	cyclobarbitone	hypnotic
Phenergan	promethazine	antihistamine

Phospholine	ecothiopate	glaucoma
Physeptone	methadone	analgesic
Picolax	sodium picosulphate	laxative
Pimafucin	natamycin	antibiotic
Pipril	piperacillin	antibiotic
Piptal	pipenzolate	antispasmodic
Piriton	chlorpheniramine	antihistamine
Pitocin	oxytocin	induction of labour
Plaquenil	hydroxychloroquine	antimalarial
Ponderax	fenfluramine	appetite depressant
Pondocillin	pivampicillin	antibiotic
Ponstan	mefenamic acid	antirheumatic
Praxilene	naftidrofuryl	vasodilator
Precortisyl	prednisolone	corticosteroid
Prednesol	prednisolone	corticosteroid
Priadel	lithium carbonate	mania
Primalan	mequitazine	antihistamine
Primolut N	norethisterone	progestogen
Primperan	metoclopramide	anti-emetic
Priscol	tolazoline	vasodilator
Pro-Banthine	propantheline	anticholinergic
Proluton-Depot	hydroxyprogesterone	progestogen
Prominal	methylphenobarbitone	epilepsy
Prondol	iprindole	antidepressant
Pronestyl	procainamide	myocardial depressant
Propaderm	beclomethasone	corticosteroid
Prostigmin	neostigmine	myasthenia

Proprietary Name	Approved Name	Main Action, Type of Drug or Use
Prostin E₂	dinoprostone	uterine stimulant
Prothiaden	dothiepin	antidepressant
Provera	medoxyprogesterone	progestogen
Pro-Viron	mesterolone	androgen
Pulmadil	rimiterol	bronchodilator
Puri-Nethol	mercaptopurine	antineoplastic
Pyopen	carbenicillin	antibiotic
Pyridium	phenazopyridine	urinary analgesic
Questran	cholestyramine	bile acid sequestrant
Rastinon	tolbutamide	oral hypoglycaemic
Razoxin	razoxane	antineoplastic
Redeptin	fluspiriline	tranquilliser
Rehibin	cyclofenil	infertility
Rheumox	azapropazone	antirheumatic
Rifadin	rifampicin	tuberculosis
Rimactane	rifampicin	tuberculosis
Ritalin	methyl phenidate	central stimulant
Rivotril	clonazepam	anticonvulsant
Robaxin	methocarbamol	muscle relaxant
Rocaltrol	calcitriol	vitamin D deficiency
Roccal	benzalkonium	antiseptic
Rogitine	phentolamine	adrenaline antagonist
Rondomycin	methacycline	antibiotic
Ronicol	nicotinyl alcohol	vasodilator
Ronyl	pemoline	cerebral stimulant

Rythmodan	disopyramide	anti-arrhythmic
Salazopyrin	sulphasalazine	sulphonamide
Saluric	chlorothiazide	diuretic
Sanomigran	pizotifen	migraine
Saroten	amitriptyline	antidepressant
Saventrine	isoprenaline	bronchodilator
Scoline	suxamethonium	muscle relaxant
Seconal	quinalbarbitone	hypnotic
Sectral	acebutolol	adrenergic blockade
Securopen	azlocillin	antibiotic
Selexid	pivmecillinam	antibiotic
Selexidin	mecillinam	antibiotic
Serc	betahistine	Ménière's disease
Serenace	haloperidol	tranquilliser
Serenid	oxazepam	tranquilliser
Serophene	clomiphene	infertility
Serpasil	reserpine	antihypertensive
Silbephylline	diprophylline	bronchodilator
Sintisone	prednisolone	corticosteroid
Sinthrome	nicoumalone	anticoagulant
Soframycin	framycetin	antibiotic
Soneryl	butobarbitone	hypnotic
Sorbitrate	isosorbide dinitrate	angina
Sotacor	sotalol	adrenergic blockade
Sparine	promazine	tranquilliser
Spiroctan	spironolactone	diuretic
Stadol	butorphanol	analgesic

Proprietary Name	Approved Name	Main Action, Type of Drug or Use
Stelazine	trifluoperazine	tranquilliser
Stemetil	prochlorperazine	tranquilliser; anti-emetic
Stromba	stanozolol	anabolic steroid
Stugeron	cinnarizine	anti-emetic
Sublimaze	fentanyl	analgesic
Sulphamezathine	sulphadimidine	sulphonamide
Surmontil	trimipramine	antidepressant
Symmetrel	amantadine	parkinsonism
Sympatol	oxedrine	vasoconstrictor
Synacthen	tetracosactrin	corticotrophin
Synadrin	prenylamine	coronary dilator
Synalar	fluocinolone	corticosteroid
Syraprim	trimethaprim	antibacterial
Synkavit	menadiol	hypoprothrombinaemia
Syntaris	flunisolide	rhinitis
Sytron	sodium ironedetate	anti-anaemic
Tace	chlorotrianisene	oestrogen
Tachyrol	dihydrotachysterol	hypocalcaemia
Tacitin	benzoctamine	tranquilliser
Tagamet	cimetidine	gastric ulcer
Talpen	talampicillin	antibiotic
Tanderil	oxyphenbutazone	antirheumatic
Taractan	chlorprothixene	tranquilliser
Tavegil	clemastine	antihistamine
Tegretol	carbamazepine	anticonvulsant, analgesic

Telepaque	iopanoic acid	contrast agent
Temgesic	buprenorphine	analgesic
Tenormin	atenolol	hypertension
Tensilon	edrophonium	anticholinesterase
Tenuate	diethylpropion	appetite depressant
Teronac	mazindol	appetite depressant
Terramycin	oxytetracycline	antibiotic
Tertroxin	liothyronine	hormone
Tetracyn	tetracycline	antibiotic
Tetralysal	lymecycline	antibiotic
Thalazole	phthalylsulphathiazole	sulphonamide
Thephorin	phenindamine	antihistamine
Thiazamide	sulphathiazole	sulphonamide
Ticar	ticarcillin	antibiotic
Tigason	etretinate	psoriasis
Tiglyssin	tigloidine	spasmolytic
Tofranil	imipramine	antidepressant
Tolanase	tolazamide	oral hypoglycaemic
Tolectin	tolmetin	antirheumatic
Tonocard	tocainide	anti-arrhythmic
Topilar	fluclorolone	corticosteroid
Torecan	thiethylperazine	anti-emetic
Tosmilen	demecarium bromide	glaucoma
Trancopal	chlormezanone	tranquilliser
Trandate	labetalol	hypertension
Tranxene	clorazepate	tranquilliser
Trasicor	oxprenolol	adrenergic blockade

Proprietary Name	Approved Name	Main Action, Type of Drug or Use
Trasylol	aprotinin	enzyme inhibitor
Tremonil	methixene	parkinsonism
Trental	oxypentifylline	bronchodilator
Trescatyl	ethionamide	tuberculosis
Trevintix	prothionamide	tuberculosis
Tridione	troxidone	anticonvulsant
Triludan	terfenadine	antihistamine
Trimopan	trimethoprim	antibacterial
Trobicin	spectinomycin	antibiotic
Tryptizol	amitriptyline	antidepressant
Tubarine	tubocurarine	muscle relaxant
Ubretid	dystigmine	anticholinesterase
Ukidan	urokinase	thrombolytic
Ultracortenol	prednisolone	corticosteroid
Ultralanum	fluocortolone	corticosteroid
Urispas	flavoxate	antispasmodic
Urolucosil	sulphamethizole	sulphonamide
Uticillin	carfecillin	antibiotic
Uvistat	mexenone	sun screen
Valium	diazepam	tranquilliser
Vallergan	trimeprazine	antihistamine
Valoid	cyclizine	anti-emetic
Vancocin	vancomycin	antibiotic
Varbian	prenalterol	B₁-adrenoceptor stimulant
Vascardin	isosorbide dinitrate	angina

Vasculit	bamethan	vasodilator
Vatensol	guanoclor	antihypertensive
Velbe	vinblastine	antineoplastic
Velosef	cephradine	antibiotic
Ventolin	salbutamol	bronchodilator
Vepesid	etoposide	antineoplastic
Vermox	mebendazole	anthelmintic
Vertigon	prochlorperazine	vertigo
Vibramycin	doxycycline	antibiotic
Vira-A	vidarabine	antineoplastic
Visclair	methylcysteine	mucolytic
Visken	pindolol	coronary dilator
Vivalan	viloxazine	antidepressant
Volital	pemoline	cerebral stimulant
Voltarol	diclofenac	antirheumatic
Welldorm	dichloralphenazone	hypnotic
Xylocaine	lignocaine	anaesthetic
Xylocard	lignocaine	anti-arrhythmic
Xylotox	lignocaine	anaesthetic
Yomesan	niclosamide	anthelmintic
Yutopar	ritodrine	premature labour
Zaditen	ketotifen	anti-asthmatic
Zantac	ranitidine	peptic ulcer
Zarontin	ethosuximide	anticonvulsant
Zelmid	zimelidine	antidepressant
Zinacef	cefuroxime	antibiotic
Zinamide	pyrazinamide	tuberculosis

Proprietary Name	Approved Name	Main Action, Type of Drug or Use
Zomax	zomepirac	analgesic
Zovirax	acyclovir	antiviral agent
Zyloric	allopurinol	uricosuric